Transformational Eldercare From The Inside Out:
Strengths-Based Strategies For Caring

James Douglas Henry
and Linda Gambee Henry

D1602583

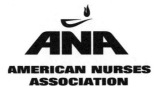

**AMERICAN NURSES
ASSOCIATION**

SILVER SPRING, MARYLAND
2007

Library of Congress Cataloging-in-Publication Data

Henry, James Douglas.
   Transformational eldercare from the inside out : strengths-based strategies for caring / James Douglas Henry and Linda Gambee Henry.
      p. ; cm.
   Includes bibliographical references and index.
   ISBN-13: 978-1-55810-229-3 (pbk.)
   ISBN-10: 1-55810-229-9 (pbk.)
      1. Community health services for older people.   2. Caregivers.   3. Older people—Services for.   4. Older people—Health and hygiene.   5. Older people—Medical care.   I. Henry, Linda Gambee.   II. Title.
   [DNLM: 1. Health Services for the Aged. 2. Aging. 3. Caregivers. 4. Geriatric Nursing. WT 31 H522t 2007]

RA564.8.T7344 2007
362'.0425—dc22   2006031405

The opinions in this book reflect those of the authors and do not necessarily reflect positions or policies of the American Nurses Association. Furthermore, the information in this book should not be construed as legal or professional advice.

ANA is the only full-service professional organization representing the nation's 2.7 million Registered Nurses through its 54 constituent member associations. ANA advances the nursing profession by fostering high standards of nursing practice, promoting the economic and general welfare of nurses in the workplace, projecting a positive and realistic view of nursing, and lobbying the Congress and regulatory agencies on healthcare issues affecting nurses and the public.

Published by
Nursesbooks.org
The Publishing Program of ANA
American Nurses Association
8515 Georgia Avenue, Suite 400
Silver Spring, MD 20910-3492
1-800-274-4ANA
http://www.nursesbooks.org/

Design and composition:
House of Equations, Inc., Arden, NC

Editing:
Lisa Munsat Anthony, Chapel Hill, NC

Indexing:
Gina Wiatrowski, Grammarians, Inc., Alexandria, VA

ISBN-13: 978-1-55810-229-3   ISBN-10: 1-55810-229-4   SAN: 851-3481

06EDIO   2.5M   10/06
First printing October 2006.

What They're Saying About Transformational Eldercare From The Inside Out

Jim and Linda Henry weave existing threads of innovative geriatric care concepts and practices into a resource tapestry that offers the knowledge and vision required for enlightened services. Through stories and an engaging writing style, the authors enable the reader to absorb facts and principles easily and enjoyably. A surprisingly wide and diverse group of topics are presented. The Henrys have again used their writing gifts and creativity to contribute a resource to the healthcare community that is indeed unique and timely.

> Charlotte Eliopoulos RN, MPH, ND, PhD
> Specialist in Holistic Geriatric and Chronic Care
> Editor, *Health Ministry Journal*

Linda and Jim Henry have combined theoretical clarity and inspirational stories that illustrate many creative and practical ways that people in the real world are transforming eldercare. This book encourages and empowers us as practitioners as it enriches us as individuals to be more person-centered and strengths-based in our work and in our lives.

> Judah L. Ronch, PhD
> VP of Resident Life, Mental Health and Wellness
> Erickson Retirement, Catonsville, MD
> Co-Editor, *Mental Wellness in Aging, Strengths-Based Approaches*

Offer[ing] an amazing but real-life array of bold new ideas, attitudes, and paradigms on a host of issues, including health care, emergency room medicine, housing, eldercare, geriatric education, spirituality, and others. It's a "must read" for professionals in the aging field who want to think more creatively about their older clients—and age more successfully themselves.

> Liz Taylor
> *Seattle Times* syndicated columnist
> Consultant and speaker on aging issues

A unique compilation of understanding the changes of aging (physiological, psychological, and spiritual) and personal vignettes. The separate discourses and portrayals provide a rich tapestry for thinking about aging in an intimate and introspective manner. A compelling introduction to the field of aging and also a refreshing look at aging for those who have been in the field for a while.

> Ruth F. Craven, EdD, RN, BC, FAAN
> Professor, Biobehavioral Nursing and Health Systems
> Associate Dean for Educational Innovations
> University of Washington School of Nursing

As eldercare laboriously undergoes a much-needed transformation, the preponderance of choices can become daunting. Jim and Linda Henry have explored the theories, concepts, and models of care in this field [and] lend credence and honor to the growing number of scholars, practitioners, and individuals who see the beauty and continued growth possible during elderhood. The reader is left with much to ponder and with a comprehensive array of resources for further exploration.

> Sandy Ransom, RN, MSHP
> Vice-President,
> Eden Alternative™ Board

James and Linda Henry's timely and clear call for a transformation in eldercare constitutes a challenge that must be met. Through exciting, enlightening, and insightful stories of professionals and practitioners in varying disciplines, one catches the spirit of a new way of eldercare that leads one to ask why change to more humane and fulfilling caregiving seems so difficult. The creative and nurturing examples of approaches to aging and caregiving offer hope that aging and sharing an elder's journey can be a time of mutual discovery, fulfillment, and growth.

> The Reverend Earl E. Shelp, PhD
> President and Co-Founder, Interfaith CarePartners®

[This book] brings together, in an intimate and engaging way, some of the most experienced and respected voices currently at work in the fields of aging and long-term care [in] an altogether valuable and inspiring book. It is valuable because it offers many new ideas for practice that are the product of the creative thinking and on-the-ground experience of experts in our field; it is inspiring because, through the commitment to caring we witness in these extraordinary individuals, we and our own work are enriched.

> Michele Mathes, JD
> Director, Education and Training
> Center for Advocacy for the Rights and Interests of the Elderly

The Henrys' book is filled with an understanding of what it means to grow older and to care for those who are aging. From a variety of cultural perspectives, it reminds all of us to relate to ourselves and others with respect, kindness, empathy, and love. The true stories from caregivers will inspire and provide models to be emulated by concerned and informed healthcare professionals

> Kathleen Sanford, RN, DBA
> Nurse Executive, author of *Leading With Love*
> Nurse Consultant; Healthcare Columnist; Healthcare Executive

Dedication

We dedicate this book to Jim's sister Barbara and her husband, Frank Davis, Jr. whose tragic, untimely deaths further validate the urgency for transformational eldercare.

Contents

Acknowledgments   xi

Introduction: The Transformations Within Transformational Eldercare   xiii
    Why This Book?   xv
    The Interviews: Perspective and Methodology   xvi
    Overview of the Book   xvii
    Transformational Strategies and Resources at a Glance   xx
    Other Strategies and Resources   xxiii

References   xxiv

Acronyms in Eldercare   xxv

Section 1   Current Realities Of Aging and Their Transformation

Aging and Elderhood in Today's Society   3
    What is Real About Aging?   3
        Why Transformational Eldercare? Some Statistics   4
        Aging in Contemporary America—An Overview   5
        Some Facts About Aging in America   6
        Ageism and Elder Stereotyping   7
    Four Models of Aging   10
        The Diminishment Model   11
        The Leisure Model   11
        The Achievement Model   12
        The Spiritual Growth Model   13

The Worth of Elders: What Will They Be Good For?   15

Being and Doing: Two Intertwining Ways   15

Characteristics of Being and Doing   17

Elders as Masters of Balance: Being and Doing United   19

Eden Alternative™: A Transformational Approach to Eldercare   19

Gerotranscendence: A Transformational Philosophy of Aging   20

The Worth of Elders: What *Are* They Good For?   22

References   25

Section 2   Emerging Innovative Caring Concepts

BUILDING A NEW GERIATRIC EMERGENCY MEDICINE SUBSPECIALTY   29
Neal Flomenbaum, MD, FACP, FACEP, and Michael Stern, MD

ENHANCING ELDER LIFE IN HOSPITALS   36
Sharon K. Inouye, MD, MPH

MERCY HEALTH CENTER   40
Christine H. Weigel, RN, BSN, MBA

LOOKING FOR THE GAPS IN ELDERCARE   43
Suyrea Reynolds, NHA

CARRIER OF THE LIGHT IN HOSPICE CARE   46
Donna Brook, RN

BRIDGING TROUBLED WATERS   51
Nancy Merrill, Improving Care Program Assistant

WEAVING A TAPESTRY OF HEALTHCARE RESOURCES   53
Cathleen Ingle, MSW

REMEMBERING PAPAW   58
Francie Horn, LCSW, CCBT, BCD

"GOING WITH THE FLOW"—CARING FOR THE ELDERLY   62
Jocelyn Porquez, NP, CS, APRN-BC

References   66

Section 3   Emerging Eldercare Communities

LIVING LIFE IN THE GARDEN OF EDEN: SHERBROOKE COMMUNITY CENTRE   69
Suellen Beatty, MScN, MSM

KLEIN CENTER—LONG-TERM LIFE ENHANCEMENT   73
Amy Leilaini Vandiver, Life Enhancement Coordinator

TIGERPLACE   77
Marilyn Rantz, PhD, RN, FAAN

KENDAL AT ITHACA   80
Dale Corson, PhD, and Maria Giampaolo, BS, CRT

ELDERHEALTH NORTHWEST—AGING IN COMMUNITY   84
Nora Gibson, MSW, Teresa Hernandez, CNA, and Donna Bergman, BA

ADULT FAMILY HOME SETTING   90
Lisa Jackson, CNA

References   92

Section 4   Higher Education and In-House Training Programs

BUILDING GERIATRIC NURSING CAPACITY   97
Patricia D. Franklin, MSN, RN

THE JOHN A. HARTFORD FOUNDATION INSTITUTE FOR GERIATRIC NURSING AT NEW YORK
    UNIVERSITY COLLEGE OF NURSING   101
Elaine Gould, MSW

BEACON OF CARE   106
Sarah Kagan, PhD, RN

PASSIONATE NURSE EDUCATOR   110
Anne Vanderbilt, RN, MSN

GOOD SAMARITAN SOCIETY   113
Gail Blocker, LNHA

Section 5   Spirituality and Aging

SACRED AT ANY AGE   119
Rabbi Cary Kozberg

MINISTRY OF POSITIVE PRESENCE   123
Kenneth L. Nolen, MDiv

ELDER SPIRITUALITY AND CARE FOR THE COGNITIVELY IMPAIRED   127
Marty Richards, MSW

EASTERN THOUGHT AS IT RELATES TO SOULFUL AGING   132
Charles Emlet, PhD, MSW

ARCHITECT OF SACRED SPACE   136
Jim Fondriest, Pastoral Care/Bereavement Coordinator

References   139

Section 6   Wide-Ranging Innovative Resources and Testimonies

COMMUNICATING AND RESOLVING CONFLICT IN ELDER FAMILY SYSTEMS   143
John Gibson, DSW, PhD, MSW, MS

CARING FOR THE WISE ONES   148
Michelle Bowman, RN

OPTIMISTIC RAINBOW MAKER   152
Donna Oiland, Community Outreach Coordinator

LIFE REVIEW, REPAIR, AND PURPOSE   156
Julia Balzer Riley, RN, MN, AHN-BC, CET®

MONTGOMERY HOSPICE   160
Beverly Paukstis, RN, MS, CHPN, and Drew Lermond, RN

ADOPTING AN ELDER   163
Amy Brown, BSN, RN

MUSIC HEALING PRACTITIONER   167
Kathleen Masters, RN, BSN

THE HEALING POWER OF TRUST   172
Liz Hopkins, RN, C

AGING AND HIV/AIDS   174
Charles A. Emlet, PhD, ACSW

References   176

Closing Reflections   179

**Appendix: Living and Leaving a Strengths-Based Legacy:
    Life Purpose Doesn't End at Age 65 or 95   183**

Bibliography   187

Index   191

Acknowledgments

We are tremendously grateful to the many people who made this book possible. We appreciate the many people without whose interest, encouragement, and suggestions this book would not have been possible. We extend our profound thanks to all of the individuals who so graciously and enthusiastically participated, providing us with their knowledge and rich, innovative perspectives. People identified by first name are real, but the names have been changed to protect confidentiality. Our appreciation goes out to the reviewers who helped with the development from proposal to manuscript: Bolton Anthony, EdD; Sherry A. Greenberg, MSN, APRN, BC; R. Gregory LaGoy, ND; Elizabeth M. Munsat, MSN, RN, BC. We are deeply indebted to Rosanne O'Connor Roe, whose inspirational personal story and suggestions spurred us on; to our editor, Eric Wurzbacher, for his wonderful creativity and enthusiastic support; to our copy editor, Lisa Anthony, whose perfectionist's eye kept us on track; and to the ANA for once again taking a chance on a "different" kind of book.

Introduction:
The Transformations Within Transformational Eldercare

Which statement is true? This . . .

"Today older people live longer but experience physical and mental diminishment over time, leading to ill health. As financial resources diminish, many of them end up in some ghetto-like eldercare institutions experiencing loneliness, helplessness, and boredom as they wait to die."

Or this?

"Intensifying research on the processes of aging indicates that older adulthood can represent a highly desirable stage in life of social, psychological, and spiritual expansion. With their wisdom and lifetime of experience, given opportunities, elders can further develop their talents and contribute to society based on their strengths."

The answer is that both statements are true. Lilia Denmark is just one example of the second. We first met Lilia Denmark who had recently turned 103 and had just retired from her career as a pediatrician. Many of us have clear perceptions about someone of that advanced age. We envision someone who is frail, and it is a true compliment to be described as being "sharp and alert."

"I retired," she said, "because my eyesight is going." The value placed on her experience and wisdom was obvious by the frequent visits of former patients and their parents who stopped by her gracious antebellum home outside Atlanta or who phoned her for advice. "My only fear," she said emphatically, "is growing old!"

Robert, on the other hand, serves as a tragic example of the first statement. Successful, independent, and respected for most of his life, he was deteriorating physically and mentally from heart disease and depression in his late seventies.

Overmedicated and in apparent despair, his frailty, depression, and contemplation of suicide led to his placement in an institution where he refused to eat, and he died.

Lilia and Robert represent two extremes of a continuum. In reality, most elders fall somewhere in between, depending upon overall life experiences, health, beliefs, and values. Yet it is fair to say that there exists in our culture a strong undercurrent pulling us toward negative perceptions of aging. Consider the following:

- What are the predominant images of older adults as portrayed in the media? Admittedly, an increasing number of advertisements, television programs, and movies represent aging Americans more respectfully than the infamous "I can't get up" ads. However, a significant number continue portraying elders as docile, nearly passive recipients of someone's help before they can get on with their lives, silly, stubborn, and worst of all, cute. They may be seen as ugly, toothless, confused, and childish.

- Elsewhere in the popular culture of jokes and stories that circulate via e-mail and the Internet, there is a distinctive denigration of the old as simply infirm and deteriorating.

- The sheer numbers of elders who are "put out to pasture" is not a media stereotype: of the growing percentage of Americans over 65 who are committed to long-term care facilities, one questions how many really need to be there or might do better in another setting. As you will find later in this book, there is considerable argument for moving away from traditional long-term care facilities and to the development of new models.

- The reality of negativism toward the elderly and the pervasive ageism within our culture is not lost on the population in general. In a 2005 poll conducted by The PARADE/Research!America Health Poll Charlton Research Company, a cross section of one thousand Americans was asked about their attitudes toward aging and longevity. The survey showed that 62% of the respondents believe that people who are older are discriminated against in our society; 50% believe that older people are not viewed with respect (www.researchamerica.org/polldate/2005/Americans+longevity).

Perhaps because of the medical advancements allowing people to live longer, healthier lives, we often hear people hoping to "live long and die quickly." There is no denying that with age comes change with its ensuing problems, and for countless numbers of individuals, the reality is that they live long and suffer long. This fear pushes people to invest huge amounts of time and money into prolonging middle age. The cosmetic industry is booming with anti-aging products. And, as noted in Section 1 of this book, *Aging and Elderhood in Today's Society*, cosmetic plastic surgery is, if not the norm, rapidly gaining in popularity for aging women and men alike.

Ultimately, all such efforts will eventually be doomed, because our bodies *will ultimately* age. Even more regrettable, many people will develop physical, cognitive, sensory, or other disabilities that limit their ability to take care of themselves. According to the 2000 U.S. Bureau of Census, 3.1 million adults age 65 and older out of a total of 35 million live with such problems.

One of the dominant paradigms related to the aging process in our culture is the diminishment model, which tends to promote the perception that aging primarily brings a series of problems that must be managed as people experience physical and mental deterioration. Unfortunately, the modern Western medical model of reducing people to biological problems and deficits supports it.

On the other hand, based upon the theories and research associated with Erik Erikson, Jungian psychology, and gerotranscendence (to name just a few), most older adults move toward holistic elderhood in some fashion. The perspective of gerotranscendent development reconceives some behaviors as age-appropriate growth, some of which can be erroneously labeled as pathological by caregivers.

This research is highlighted in *The Worth of Elders: What Will They Be Good For?* in Section 1. In particular, some of the most recent research on gerotranscendence has been conducted by gerontologist Lars Tornstam and his team at Uppsala University in Sweden proposing an inner move toward maturation by many elders (Tornstam 2005). Swiss psychologist Carl Jung called it the process of individuation (higher level of consciousness, completion, wholeness), and developmental researcher Erik Erikson labeled it ego integrity (inner harmony, self-acceptance). In his book, *The Mature Mind*, gerontologist Gene Cohen speaks extensively of "the Inner Push," a "life force composed of many individual forces, like springtime sap rising through the myriad channels and pores inside a tree, propelling the flowering and seasonal growth" (Cohen 2005, pp. 31–32). Like the flowering tree, it pushes us toward new growth and creativity.

Why This Book?

We do not mean to discount the desire to look and feel good as one ages. We do suggest that how our culture views aging impacts everything related to aging, from retail products and services to health care. We couldn't agree more with the suggestion that the coming crisis of a dwindling supply of nursing professionals coupled with the onslaught of an aging population may be health care's perfect storm. There is no question that we must avert a health crisis precipitated by such a storm. The cultural perception of aging, both positive and negative, affects not only the delivery of all healthcare services, both inpatient and outpatient, but it also directly impacts how we as a society design living environments that promote the concept of "living until you die."

This book is designed for eldercare service providers from a variety of disciplines. "Today we have a foundational understanding of what it means to age, and it needs to be shared with almost all caregivers," states Sarah Kagan, PhD, RN, gerontological associate professor at the University of Pennsylvania School of Nursing. "Even in pediatrics, one can run into aging issues. Someone may have a grandmother caring for grandchildren because their mother is ill or working."

We believe that to change the outside world, as the discussion above represents in part, we must begin with ourselves. *We*—who are both the caretakers *and* the future elders—are the ones who need to change from the inside out in order to get to a society of individuals where holistic care might be a matter of fact. By "inside out" we mean:

- discarding outdated beliefs about elderhood;
- promoting healthy, caring elder environments through employing a variety of strategies and resources;
- assisting service providers to learn and live a caregiving legacy through the use of a variety of tools; and
- actively preparing for one's own demise.

By "strengths-based," we mean finding out what has helped the elder get this far in life and using that as the primary framework for caregiving to each elder individual. Each of us has his or her inherent talents, experiences, knowledge, values, and interests that, taken together, frame how we approach our lives. Rather than viewing a person solely as a diagnosis to be cured or a problem to be solved, the professional caregiver must connect with this unique and essential self. When we focus attention upon a person's strengths, problems loom less large (Kivnick and Murray 2001).

> *"My [elderly] clients and their families give back a thousandfold."*
> —Cathleen Ingle, MSW

The Interviews: Perspective and Methodology

Our goal was to identify emerging and innovative caring concepts related to elder healthcare delivery, eldercare communities, and geriatric education. To that end, we interviewed more than 37 nurses, social workers, chaplains, physicians, health ministers, long-term care administrators, Certified Nursing Assistants (CNAs), and nursing educators representing hundreds of thousands of dedicated eldercare professionals. They were selected based upon their specialties and upon recommendations from people interviewed for our previous books, from various organizations, and from participants of workshops we have been conducting nationally. Whenever possible, we sought geographical diversity. We wanted to dialogue with hands-on caregivers as well as noted experts in the fields of geriatrics and gerontology, eldercare management, senior service programming, and chaplaincy. As you will see from the variety of settings noted in the Table of Contents, this book does not represent an exhaustive coverage of eldercare services. Rather, it is a representative cross section of eldercare services and providers.

We believe the extraordinary stories of ordinary people working in everyday, diverse ways will expand mutual understanding, causing the reader to reflect, "That experience or belief articulates what I've been feeling for a long time." Hopefully, these stories will serve to revitalize other caregivers' passion for their professions.

We include perceptions on the nature and critical importance of spirituality in eldercare as well as the biomedical, psychological, and social services that comprise eldercare. We made every effort not to impose our personal perceptions of spirituality, allowing interviewees to shape and articulate what *spiritual* means for each of them. Whether the word is used openly or not, a healthy sense of spirituality is vital to caregiving.

Although Linda has many years of experience in healthcare education, communications, and marketing, neither of us is a geriatric specialist. Therefore, we incorporated a participatory research methodology called *action research*, a spiral process that alternates between action (in our case interviewing), critical reflection, and research.

First coined in 1947 by Kurt Lewin, a German psychologist and one of the pioneers of social psychology, action research is described by the Society and Culture Association as an informal, qualitative, interpretive, reflective, and experimental methodology that requires all the participants to be collaborative researchers. It is a spiral process of planning, acting, observing, and reflecting that is ongoing until the most desirable outcomes for all participants are achieved. We chose this approach because we believe it to be a particularly useful tool in compiling and communicating innovative eldercare information that will, hopefully, support and encourage eldercare transformation. To some extent, the information gathering and problem solving process invites us all, with profound empathy, to share in this transformation by hypothetically "growing old beforehand."

As one advocate of the method notes: "All theorists of action research offer models or cycles in which thinking, doing and watching are interwoven and repeated throughout the research activity. . . . For example, action research can be seen as a process where instructors, teachers or employees become responsible for managing the process of change within any aspect of an organization" (Taylor 2002). (For a detailed treatment of action research as such and its applications and possibilities in healthcare educational and practice settings, consult Waterman et al. 2001.)

Overview of the Book

We said that by "inside out" we mean, in part, preparing for one's inevitable demise. Many voices—across the ages and throughout these interviews—have suggested that consciously preparing for one's ultimate death and overcoming one's fear of that death frees us up for living fully and joyfully in the present. We believe the same holds true for preparing for elderhood. When caregivers more fully understand older adults, serving them holistically as well as clinically, we serve ourselves as well.

In the following pages, you will learn about the nature of elderhood, not only in terms of growing problems and diminishment, but in promoting transformational elderhood as a time of life that is also marked by social, psychological, and spiritual expansion. You will find a wide variety of strategies and resources available to care for elders which you can apply to your professional practice and/or your personal situation.

The creative insights found within this book are not limited to one theoretical school. As Gene Cohen's recent national study demonstrates, seniors actively engaged in creative activities have significantly better overall mental and physical health, as indicated by fewer falls, fewer doctor visits, less use of medications, fewer vision problems, less loneliness and depression, and an increased level of involvement in any number of activities. As he sums up his findings:

> Truly this is a creative age, for humanity and for each of us, whether we are fully retired, on the verge of retirement, or still in the prime of our young life. Our willingness to embrace the challenge and the opportunity will define the legacy that each of us builds, and the gift that each of us gives, in every season of our lives (Cohen 2000, p. 309).

The importance of training healthcare professionals to understand the unique differences aging adults present was universally emphasized in our interviews. Nursing educators were not alone in advocating an increased emphasis on geriatric training. Acknowledging the social worker's unique caregiving role and given the increasing numbers of aging clients, the National Association of Social Work established an Aging Initiative aimed at raising the awareness of the profession's broad practice scope. Additionally, there is a growing importance placed on spirituality in the lives of elders. Traditionally, the tendency has been to leave out the spiritual component, with caregivers focused primarily on the physical, social, and psychological aspects of a patient or client's life. However, leaving out the spiritual dimension is like losing one limb.

To aid in training and educational efforts, we developed a Facilitator's Guide, available on CD, as a companion to the book. Both the book and the guide are designed to integrate multiple caregiving perspectives in ways that are useful and transforming and to present a wide array of concepts and programs that healthcare professionals and educators can use immediately. The information can easily be used within a classroom setting as stand-alone sessions or as adjunct resources to current geriatric class content.

Here are highlights of some of the material you will discover in subsequent sections:

Section 1: Current Realities of Aging and Their Transformation
Basic social, economic, and demographic realities about aging in America are shared, along with some prevalent stereotypes related to getting older. Four models of aging are offered: diminishment, leisure, achievement, and spiritual growth.

The characteristics of two fundamental energies of *doing* and *being* are outlined. A growing amount of research indicates that elderhood can represent a highly desirable stage in life of expanded social, psychological, and spiritual dimensions. Five distinctive qualities of mature elderhood are delineated in response to the question, "What are elders good for?"

Section 2: Emerging Innovative Caring Concepts

Highlights include the first geriatric emergency medicine fellowship, the Hospital Elder Life Program (HELP), and several other inpatient eldercare programs designed to increase beneficial outcomes. Transitional programs to help bridge the gap between the diagnosis of a terminal illness and hospice and additional specific, more holistic caring practices are identified.

Section 3: Emerging Eldercare Communities

Transformational eldercare communities are emerging throughout the United States and internationally. Eden Alternative™ leads the way and serves as a new model for a number of more traditional long-term care facilities. Some organizations innovate by constructing new small, home-like buildings built within small community settings. Aging in community and aging in place are emerging concepts of care.

Section 4: Higher Education and In-House Training Programs

A growing number of healthcare organizations are beginning to recognize older adults as their core business. Roughly 50% of all hospital beds are filled by people 65 or older. Yet, nursing schools are only now beginning to appreciate the importance of geriatric content in their curricula. The John A. Hartford Foundation supports many of the educational innovations taking place today.

Section 5: Spirituality and Aging

Wise care providers understand that many elders embrace a sense of cosmic communion. Through numerous faith traditions, elders may experience a time of deepening spiritual awareness and growth.

Section 6: Wide-Ranging Innovative Resources and Testimonies

Many eldercare providers bring to the profession a wide range of innovative resources, just a few being music, art, Healing Touch, and life review therapies. In the process, they find themselves blessed by the many intangible gifts they receive in return from elders.

Transformational Eldercare from the Inside Out: Strategies and Resources at a Glance

Innovative Programs	WHAT IS IT?	PAGE
Hospital Elder Life Program	Cost-effective model designed to prevent hospital care of elders that can be toxic.	36–39
Transition Program	Program designed to bridge the time between a terminal diagnosis and hospice.	53–55
Improving Care Through the End of Life	Program designed to help people who are homebound to maintain their quality of life and as much independence as possible. It is a bridge assisting older patients to transition to the next level of care.	51–52
Living History Program	Process for capturing life stories.	73–74
Nurses Improving Care for Health System Elders	A program that involves gaining hospitals' commitment to providing high-quality eldercare, initiating nurse-led models of care to benefit hospitalized older patients.	102, 110–11
The Program of All-inclusive Care for the Elderly	A new benefit that features a comprehensive service delivery system and integrated Medicare and Medicaid financing, combining medical, social, and long-term care services for frail people.	116
Geriatric Resource Nurse	Acute care nurses who are certified by the American Nurses Certification Center. The goal is often to have one on every unit and every shift within the hospital.	44, 102
Adopt an Elder	Every elder has a right to have a family, which can prevent premature placement in a nursing home.	163–66
Elder Communities/Places		
Eden Alternative™	Powerful nursing home model for improving the quality of life for elders and the disabled.	19–20
Buchanan Place	Home-like residence for elders and the disabled, built from the ground up.	84–89
Greenhouse	Home-life-oriented residences designed and built especially for the disabled and elders with dementia.	89
Elder adult day health center	Model for adult day care taking components of services typically offered in a nursing home and making them available within a community.	84–85
Center on Aging and Older Adult Ministries	The arm of the United Methodist Church formed specifically to focus on ministry to elders.	13
PrestigePLUS	Wellness center model for elders.	148–51
The John A. Hartford Foundation Institute for Geriatric Nursing	Identifies, develops, and disseminates best practices in the nursing care of older adults with the focus of infusing them into the education of every nursing student and the work environment of practicing professional nurses.	98–104
Gerontological Society of America (GSA) Policy Institute	Funds and manages an elder civic engagement program.	100

Workshops/Training	WHAT IS IT?	PAGE
Honor My Wishes™	Workshop to enhance end-of-life conversations; provides personal end-of-life binder to help people organize their wishes with regard to medical care, financial affairs, and final commemorating plans. Sample forms are provided.	52
Finding Meaning in Medicine	Free resources to support healthcare groups.	56
Ethical Wills	A process for passing on personal values, beliefs, blessings, and advice to families and to future generations. www.ethicalwill.com. See also *The Legacy Center* (thelegacycenter@yahoo.com).	129
Life/Work legacy	Questions and exercise for more clearly identifying one's personal sense of legacy.	183–86
Best Nursing Practices in Care For Older Adults	Modules and a curriculum guide developed by geriatric nursing experts that provide faculty with ready-made text and audiovisuals.	102
Try This	A series of assessment instruments available to staff development educators to help them introduce defined competencies and geriatric best practices into their continuing education activities.	102, 104
Hey, I'm the Customer	Customer service training program.	74
Laughter workshops	Community workshops on the healing power of laughter and the importance of putting more humor into one's life.	154
Consumer Information		
Consumers' and Providers' Guides to Quality Care	Resources to evaluate the quality of nursing homes.	78
Observable Indicators of Nursing Home Care	Questions used to evaluate the quality of nursing homes. See http://www.nursinghomehelp.org/.	78, 144
BenefitsCheckUp	The nation's most comprehensive online service to screen for federal, state, and some local private and public benefits for older adults.	116
Human Values in Aging electronic newsletter	Published by AARP Office of Academics, it includes topics pertinent to aging.	185
Movies/Videos		
Harry and Tonto	Heart-warming movie and story of the adventuresome trip across the country of 75-year-old Harry Coombes and his cat, Tonto.	184
Wit	Based upon a play by Margaret Edson, in it Vivian Bearing becomes a hard-nosed professor who has terminal ovarian cancer. As she approaches death, she reflects upon the cycle of her cancer, the treatments, and significant events in her life.	151
Whose Life Is It Anyway?	Ken Harrison, a central character, survives a terrible car accident that leaves him paralyzed. When he decides that he wants life-saving dialysis discontinued so he can die on his own terms, his decision precipitates a medical, ethical, and legal conflict between physicians devoted to the practice of paternalistic, aggressive treatment.	151
Discovering Everyday Spirituality	Series of four videos by Thomas Moore to promote the recalling and retelling of significant life events.	82
Morrie, Lessons on Living	Video of Ted Koppel's intimate discussions with retired professor Morrie Schwartz, who was dying from Lou Gehrig's disease. Also, see the movie *Tuesdays with Morrie* in which Jack Lemon plays the part of Morrie Schwartz in the movie version of his story.	130, 134–35

continued

Therapies/Techniques	WHAT IS IT?	PAGE
T'ai Chi	An exercise involving movements of the body done in coordination with the mind and with one's respiration.	149
Music therapy	The use of music and sound within clinical settings which can facilitate one's self-healing capacities and is demonstrated to be useful in reducing stress, anxiety, and pain, nausea, and vomiting associated with chemotherapy.	167–71
Therapeutic Touch or Healing Touch	An energetic, non-invasive way to help calm people and reduce pain.	169
HIV/AIDS Guidelines for Eldercare Service Providers	Five basic guidelines.	176
Time Slips	A process whereby a group of people gathers in a circle and creates stories in response to a picture provided by a facilitator.	159
Stringing beads	A technique used in helping clients relate their life journey.	159
Myers-Briggs Type Indicator®	Instrument for determining one's strengths. A free version of it is on the Internet.	184
Transferable skills	Instrument for determining one's key skills.	184
Ayurvedic treatment	Indian-based system using herbal remedies.	49
Thought Field Therapy	Technique used to help people express difficult emotions.	61
Neuro-Emotive Technique	Method of finding and releasing energy blockages.	63–65
NAET (Nambudripad's Allergy Elimination Technique)	An allergy treatment procedure.	65
OH Cards	Tool to help people recall significant life events and to assist in storytelling.	82
Aging IQ	Questions testing one's knowledge of aging.	128
Ethnographic interviewing	A method of asking open-ended questions to capture significant life stories.	185
Elder theater group	Therapy for elders, including the cognitively impaired.	86
Social portfolio	Healthy elders need to develop a social portfolio as well as a financial portfolio, balancing individual and group efforts.	13
Philosophy/Research		
Harvard Adult Study	Highlights several key dimensions one needs to cultivate to age well.	12, 14
Gerotranscendence	Based on comprehensive research on mature elderhood, it means elders rising above the cultural demands of adulthood and moving in the direction of maturation, wisdom, and spiritual growth.	20
What elders are good for	Five basic attributes of what elders give to our culture.	22–24
What happens to people after death	Five interpretations.	121
Law of Manu	Four stages of Hindu life.	133
Stages of dying	Elisabeth Kubler-Ross's five stages of dying.	134

Other Strategies and Resources

NOTE: These strategies and resources, while not mentioned in this book, are but a sample of what we have discovered exists in the eldercare community. We would appreciate hearing from the reader about any additional items. jlhenry@aol.com.

STRATEGY/RESOURCE	WHAT IS IT?
Levin Social Network Scale	Method for evaluating one's support system.
Strangers in Good Company	Movie about a group of female elders who connected deeply with each other while stranded when their bus breaks down.
The Open Road: America Looks at Aging	Video that examines the opportunities and challenges that lie ahead for individuals and society as 77 million baby boomers near retirement age. 60 minutes. $14.96 http://www.firstrunfeatures.com/openroad.html
Aerobics, T'ai Chi, and Yoga for Seniors	Series of videos. Can be located at various Web sites via Google.
Calculate your life expectancy	Determine your life expectancy based upon factors such as genes, health, environment, etc. Go to www.nmfn.com/tn/listpages—calculator_list_pg.
Children's books on aging	A list of 91 books that depict elders in a positive light. www.gwumc.edu/cahn/booklist/index.htm.
Dance therapy	In the 2003 study reported in the New England Journal of Medicine that tracked older people in a range of leisure activities, dance was the only physical leisure activity that correlated with a decreased likelihood of the onset of dementia.
Elder circles	Small group process based upon Native American tradition of sharing wisdom.
Eldershire™	An Eldershire™ community improves the quality of life for people of all ages by strengthening and improving the means by which the community protects, sustains, and nurtures its elders. www.eldershire.net.
Hospital-At-Home	New program being piloted in several places around the country. Johns Hopkins has been developing the model since 1994. Research indicates that many hospitalized elders could be treated just as safely and effectively in their homes, and at-home care may be less expensive than in-hospital care.
Care Team® training	Offered through Interfaith Care partners in Houston. www.interfaithcarepartners.org.
Almost Home film	The Almost Home film takes you inside the revolutionary transformation of a nursing home. This companion Web site pulls back to give you the bigger picture. www.almosthomedoc.org
Elderhostel Institute Network	The Elderhostel Institute Network (EIN) is a voluntary association of Lifelong Learning Institutes (LLIs), funded by Elderhostel, Inc., a not-for-profit organization dedicated to providing educational opportunities for older adults. www.elderhostel.org
Senior Corps	Senior Corps connects today's over-55s with the people and organizations that need them most. Helps them become mentors, coaches, or companions to people in need, or contribute their job skills and expertise to community projects and organizations. www.seniorcorps.org
National Center for Creative Aging	The National Center for Creative Aging (NCCA) is dedicated to fostering an understanding of the vital relationship between creative expression and the quality of life of older people. www.creativeaging.org
AARP Resource Guide	Browse or research AARP's database on Internet resources and link to more than 900 of the best sites for people age 50+. www.aarp.org/internetresources
Center for Advocacy for the Rights and Interests of the Elderly (CARIE)	A non-profit organization based in Philadelphia dedicated to improving the quality of life for vulnerable elders.

References

Cohen, G. 2000. *The Creative Age: Awakening Human Potential in the Second Half of Life.* New York: Avon Books.

Cohen, G. 2005. *The Mature Mind.* NY: Basic Books.

Kivnick, H. & S. Murray. 2001. Life strengths interview guide: Assessing elder clients' strengths. *Journal of Gerontological Social Work* 34(4):7–31.

Taylor, M. 2002. *Action Research In Workplace Education: A Handbook For Literacy Instructors.* Ottawa: Partnerships In Learning. http://www.nald.ca/CLR/action/cover.htm (accessed July 30, 2006).

Tornstam, L. 2005. *Gerotranscendence.* New York: Springer Publishing Company.

Waterman, H., D. Tillen, R. Dickson & K. de Koning. Action research: A systematic review and guidance for assessment. *Health Technology Assessment* 2001:5(23). http://www.ncbi.nlm.nih.gov/entrez/query.fcgi?cmd=Retrieve&db=pubmed&list_uids=11785749&dopt=Citation (accessed July 30, 2006).

Acronyms in Eldercare

Since the many professionals that comprise the eldercare community come from numerous disciplines, we thought it would be useful for everyone to know the unavoidable acronyms that are used within and across those disciplines.

ACGME	Accreditation Council for Graduate Medical Education
ACSW	Academy of Certified Social Workers (certification)
AHN-BC	American Holistic Nurses, Board Certified
AIT	Administrator in Training Program
ANA	American Nurses Association
ANCC	American Nurses Credentialing Center
APRN-BC	Advanced Practice Registered Nurse, Board Certified
BA	Bachelor of Arts
BC	Board Certified
BCD	Board Certified Diplomate
BS	Bachelor of Science
BSN	Bachelor of Science in Nursing
CCBT	Certified Cognitive-Behavioral therapist
CHPN	Certified Hospice and Palliative Nurse
CET®	Certified Expressive Therapist
CNA	Certified Nursing Assistant
CS	Certified Specialist
CTRS	Certified Therapeutic Recreational Specialist
DSW	Doctorate in Social Work
ED	Emergency Department
EdD	Doctorate in Education
EM	Emergency Medicine
FAAN	Fellow of the American Academy of Nursing

FACEP	Fellow of the American College of Emergency Physicians
FACP	Fellow of the American College of Physicians
HCO	health care organization
HMO	health maintenance organization
HRSA	Health Resources and Services Administration
JCAHO	Joint Commission on Accreditation of Healthcare Organizations
LCSW	Licensed Clinical Social Worker
LLI	Lifelong Learning Institute
LNHA	Licensed Nursing Home Administrator
LPN	Licensed Practical Nurse
MBA	Master's in Business Administration
MDiv	Master of Divinity
MN	Master's in Nursing
MPH	Master's of Public Health
MS	Master's of Science
MSM	Master's of Science in Management
MSN	Master's of Science in Nursing
MScN	Master's of Science in Nursing
MSW	Master's in Social Work
NHA	Nursing Home Administrator
NP	Nurse Practitioner
POES	Physician order entry system
RN	Registered Nurse

Section 1

Current Realities of Aging and Their Transformation

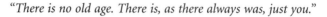

"There is no old age. There is, as there always was, just you."

—Carol Matthau
O Magazine, October 2003

In This Section . . . Aging and Elderhood in Today's Society, The Worth of Elders: What Will They Be Good For?, and The Worth of Elders: What Are They Good For?

- Aging and Elderhood in Today's Society—Basic social, economic, and demographic realities about aging in America are shared, along with some prevalent stereotypes related to getting older. . . . Four models of aging are also offered: diminishment, leisure, achievement, and spiritual growth.
- The Worth of Elders: What Will They Be Good For?—The characteristics of two fundamental energies of doing and being are outlined. . . . A growing amount of research indicates that elderhood can represent a highly desirable stage in life of expanded social, psychological, and spiritual dimensions.
- The Worth of Elders: What Are They Good For?—Five distinctive qualities of mature elderhood are delineated in response to the question, "What are elders good for?"

Aging and Elderhood in Today's Society

What is Real About Aging?

In a timeless children's tale, the Velveteen Rabbit, who is the newest arrival in the nursery, asks a question of the Skin Horse, the oldest and most play-worn of the toys:

> "What is REAL?" asked the Rabbit one day. "Does it mean having things that buzz inside you and a stick-out handle?" "Real isn't how you are made," said the Skin Horse. "It's a thing that happens to you. When a child loves you for a long, long time, not just to play with, but REALLY loves you, then you become Real. It doesn't happen all at once. You become. It takes a long time. Generally, by the time you are Real, most of your hair has been loved off, and your eyes drop out and you get loose in the joints and very shabby. But these things don't matter at all, because once you are Real you can't be ugly, except to people who don't understand" (Williams 1922).

What is real for aging adults in America's twenty-first century? The answer is different for each individual. The complexities related to growing older are as broad and diverse as are elders and their individual situations, as seen in the two examples of Lilia and Robert in the Introduction. We would be remiss if we did not acknowledge the health and financial challenges facing many elders.

When Jessie's mother began demonstrating signs of dementia several years ago, her family didn't fully realize what was happening. "My mother always was a difficult person to get along with and I suspect was a little emotionally disturbed," Jessie recounts. The encroaching dementia behaviors were viewed as being "just more" of her strangeness. As the stages progressed, however, it became apparent that the progression was related to a physical problem. Even though Jessie's father had some physical difficulties and was not really physically able to care for his wife, he was unwilling to seek other residential care. Coping with the enormity of what the family faced fell to Jessie and her siblings.

"Neither my sister, who lives in another community, nor my brother is available to help; so I've really assumed the role of information gatherer, learning about what resources there are and providing hands-on care of my mother for periods of time so my father can get a break. I find it interesting that of the children, I was the one as a teenager and young adult who was more rebellious and didn't get along with my mother, and now I'm the one guiding her care.

"My mother seldom talks now but seems to enjoy the facials that I give her. One of the most troubling new behaviors that I just don't know how to deal with is my mother's problems related to toileting herself. Even though we make certain that she doesn't get constipated, she tries to reach back and extract her feces as she is having a bowel movement. I didn't realize that was happening until I took her to the bathroom the other day. I don't know how long this has been going on, but earlier I had noticed brownish streaks on walls and assumed it was dirt."

Jessie found a referral to a geriatric psychiatrist very helpful in managing her mother's illness and in dealing with her father's denial of the severity of the dementia. "The psychiatrist found Mom to be in the advanced stages of dementia. The antipsychotic medication he prescribed has made enormous difference in relieving her episodes of violence that were triggered by huge irritations in her environment. For example, she might become angry if someone were wearing earrings or was fat."

Jessie looks forward to working with a new case manager who will help the family negotiate the maze of available services. "I know my mother needs to be placed now in a residential facility, but my father is not ready to take that step. In the interim, we take my mother to a wonderful day health facility three days a week. This allows my father to have care of my mother for periods of time so my father can get a break."

Why Transformational Eldercare? Some Statistics

Jessie and her family are not alone in trying to cope with the realities that some elder families face and the costs associated with that care. According to Judith Feder, veteran health policy analyst and dean of Georgetown University's Public Policy Institute in Washington, DC, only about 1.6 million elders are in nursing homes. Of that number, about one million are on Medicaid. She notes that projections of people currently retiring indicate that about 30% are likely to die without ever needing long-term care, fewer than 17% are likely to need one year of care or less, and about 20% are likely to need care for more than five years (Feder 2005). She is not alone in suggesting that, while the need may be unpredictable, the consequences can be catastrophic. Feder further asserts that research at Georgetown and elsewhere reveals that most elder people lack the financial resources to pay for extended nursing home care.

Two out of three seniors rely on Medicaid to cover nursing home bills, and by the time boomers are fully assimilated into the ranks of the aged in 2040, $760 billion will be spent per year on their long-term care needs from all sources. Congress hopes to cut $10 billion from Medicaid by 2010 (Sloane 2005). The impact on eldercare is potentially huge, depending on how much funding is eventually cut.

The financial implications related to health care and other services for an aging population are undeniable. The consequences to their quality of life are enormous. This book is not meant to suggest ways of solving the current financial dilemma. That it must be solved is clear, and those wiser than us will do it. Our intent is not to gloss over the realities faced by some families. Rather, our purpose is to invite providers of service and others to consider new and different concepts and models of caring. Caring for an aging society does not have to remain the same. We, among others, believe that reinventing the future for an elder society not only is possible but has begun.

Regardless of how old we are, we all are involved in the process of aging. There is no "they and we." The more we know about this process and embrace our own aging, the more we can reclaim the energy that often goes into fear and denial and use it more constructively. Death itself is normal, natural, and necessary.

The terms *older adult, senior citizen, and elder* are often used interchangeably. The definition of an older person varies from 65 and older (as used by the federal government) to "someone who is older than I am." One way of categorizing aging is: young–old (65–74), old–old, (75–84), oldest–old (85-plus). "Perhaps, we should start referring to the elderly as 'experienced adults,'" suggests Neal Flomenbaum, MD, Emergency Physician-in-Chief at New York-Presbyterian Hospital, Weill Cornell Medical Center, who heads a new, first-of-its-kind geriatric emergency medicine fellowship.

> *"Death is absolutely safe. Nobody every fails it."*
> — Ram Dass
> *Still Here: Embracing Aging, Changing and Dying*

In this book, we define an elder as "a person over the age of 65 who is moving toward maturation, wisdom, and spiritual growth." We acknowledge that the use of age 65 to define elderhood is outdated, but we choose to use it until the norm is changed.

Arguably, many eldercare institutions remain in dire need of transformation. Some interviewees for this book claim that these institutions are a combination of a hospital and a poorhouse, elderly ghettos. And, the frequently over-worked staff may withdraw behind what has been called the "Berlin Wall." An "I-Thou" mentality of treating each person as valued for his/her humanity appears absent in many eldercare institutions. And, society views older adults—especially those in institutions—as somehow different, apart from, and less than the rest of the human race (Ronch & Goldfield 2003).

There are a number of individuals, groups, and organizations already committed to transforming eldercare. To name just a few organizations so dedicated, we note Eden Alternative™, ElderHealth Northwest, TigerPlace, and the Hospital Elder Life Program (HELP), the latter of which has been implemented in more than 50 health-care organizations. If any of these are new to you, this book will introduce you to them and to the ideas and ideals in which they are grounded.

Aging in Contemporary America—An Overview

"What is old?" asks Sarah H. Kagan, Associate Professor and Doris R. Schwartz Term Professor in Gerontological Nursing at the University of Pennsylvania School of

Nursing. "Except for those who may suffer from a chronic condition or disease, the general perception is that someone in their sixties or early seventies is really not old," she states. "Many people can't give a particularly apt definition of what is old, which I believe represents a kind of crossroads in our society. Toward that end, I am very optimistic that we are in a time of flux where people are reevaluating their perceptions about aging."

We agree wholeheartedly with those who believe that all older people are vital human beings and that having a physical or mental impairment due to aging does not diminish adequacy and worth. As Amy Brown, BSN, RN, who with her partner adopted Marilyn, an elderly friend with dementia, put it, "I believe that all elderly people are vitally important. . . . They are human beings with essence and deserve our respect and gratitude. Even with her disease, Marilyn has spirit and real meaning, threads of which come through even in the most difficult of circumstances; that is what we are spending our time with."

It is true that people age at a different pace, and age and disease are not synonymous. U.S. Bureau of Census (2000) statistics tell us that at any given time, only 5% of the elderly reside in nursing homes, although roughly 50% of them will be residents at some point in their lives. As the brief discussion in the following section indicates, however, there are a great number of elder Americans, whatever their state of dependence.

Some Facts About Aging in America

The economic impact of a growing population 50 years and older is huge. Consider: Individuals who are 50 years and older represent a segment of the population that is growing three times faster than the overall population. They represented 25% of the population in 2004, controlled 77% of the nation's assets, accounted for 40% of consumer demand, and had a median net worth of $188,500 in 2004. Women comprise 75% of the older poor (Hooyman & Kiyak 2004).

Ken Dychtwald tells us, in *Age Power: How the 21ˢᵗ Century Will Be Ruled by the New Old*, that one-third of the boomers will be able to retire at age 65; one-third will need to work to age 70 before having sufficient funds to retire; and one-third will never be able to retire if they don't want to live in poverty (Dychtwald 1999, p. 7). Although statistics may vary, the consensus is that many baby boomers will be unable to retire.

In 1990, persons aged 55 and older represented 27% of the labor force (U.S. Census 1990). The U.S. Bureau of Labor Statistics (Cohen 2000) projected the following breakdown of labor force participation in 2005:

> *More Facts*
>
> - 76 million baby boomers
> - Nearly 8,000 turning 60 each day
> - By 2030, 25% of population will be 60+
> - 85+ is the fastest growing age group
> - 85% of women outlive their husbands
>
> Source: U.S. Census Bureau Fact Finder. http://factfinder.census.gov.

- Men 55–64   67.9%
- Men 65-plus   16.0%
- Women 55–64   54.3%
- Women 65-plus   8.8%

Even churches must be attuned to ministering to older adults. Often programming objectives are geared toward young families with children. However, it is estimated for every young adult under 25 years old within a church, there are six senior citizens 65 years or older (Sauer 2005, p. 7).

Ageism and Elder Stereotyping

Our culture embraces a gerontophobic fear—implying that the worse thing that can happen to you is to look and grow old. In fact, a February 1, 2002 news release from the American Society for Aesthetic Plastic Surgery (ASAPS), noted the increase in cosmetic surgery procedures on older adults. Compiled statistics revealed that that 7% of cosmetic procedures performed in 2000 were done on women and men age 65 and older. Since 1997, the number of cosmetic procedures performed on people in this age group increased by 352% (*AORN Journal* 2002) (http://www.surgery.org). [Authors' note: Per ASAPS release, no author noted but asks for statistical credit go to the ASAPS.] Notes Malcolm Paul, MD, a past president of ASAPS, "People today see no reason to age in the traditional way. They want to look their best at every age, and cosmetic surgery can help them do that." Overall, according to statistics compiled by the American Society of Plastic Surgeons, Americans spent $12.4 billion in 2004 on plastic surgery. While women account for 87% of all cosmetic surgery, the number of men undergoing cosmetic surgery increased to 1.2 million men in 2004. Men appear to view cosmetic surgery as a way of looking more youthful in a competitive work world.

Ageism in our culture is similar to sexism and racism. The longer we live, the longer we are impacted by negative stereotypes of the elderly. Old is a bad word. AARP (American Association of Retired Persons) and terms like *prime timers* and *senior citizens* are substitutes. Dr. Flomenbaum observes, "Whenever you use the words 'elderly', 'geriatrics', 'senior citizen,' or any of the current euphemisms or substitute words, you almost always see a frown on someone's face." Robert Butler, MD, first defined ageism in 1969 as a "deep-seated uneasiness on the part of the young and middle-aged—a personal revulsion to and distaste for growing old, disease, disability; and fear of powerlessness, 'uselessness' and death" (Butler 1969).

"If you open your children's schoolbooks and look in the index under 'aging' or 'elderly', what will you find? Nothing" (Dychtwald 1999). From the height of steps in public buildings to the time it takes for traffic lights to change, our physical environment is designed for youth and younger adults.

Gene Cohen, MD, PhD, Director of the Center on Aging, Health and Humanities at George Washington University, suggests that there may be a cultural belief that at a certain age it is appropriate for old people to do society a favor and disappear from the landscape. He relates the story of a meeting to defend a budget request for research studies of aging and diseases of later life. One congressman was critical of spending money on these studies because he felt it represented an inequitable distribution of dollars for the elderly, suggesting that adopting a "historical" perspective, which would put greater resources into health care for the young and allow "nature to take its course," would be a better approach (Cohen 2000).

In the course of writing this book, almost without exception, caregivers and educators emphasized the importance of understanding the aging process and examining our perceptions of aging. What are our own perceptions related to getting older, and what stereotypes can we identify? Some of the most prevalent stereotypes are listed below.

People over 65 are old.

Career counselor, Helen Harkness, PhD, asserts that it is not how old you are, but how old you think you are and how old you function that is important. She suggests that the period between age 60 and 80 is more of a *second midlife* than it is a time for retirement and diminished achievement (Harkness 1999). This is not as unrealistic as it may seem considering that, barring disease, accidents, and environmental and lifestyle factors, the life span of a human is about 120 years. Ken Dychtwald believes that "using 65 as a marker of old age—and the onset of old-age entitlements—is meaningless, unfair, and even dangerous" (Dychtwald 1999).

Older people are pretty much the same.

An older woman laments, "When people look at me and see someone who is older and gray haired, they don't look again." Actually, older people are as diverse as any other group and age physically, mentally, and emotionally at a varying pace, influenced by genetic, environmental, and lifestyle factors. If you encounter one older person, you've encountered one older person.

Dr. Flomenbaum states, "Chronological age should not be the major criterion in how we view elders. I like to use the analogy of a vintage car; we all know of older cars that have been well cared for, are attractive, and still run fine. On the other hand, there are newer cars that have been neglected and, as a result, don't run well at all. I think that how people age is a combination of lifestyle, how they have maintained their health, and their genetics. These factors are often more important than whether someone is 73 or 83."

Older people don't change.

The folly of this belief is exposed by the reality that people, older or otherwise, who don't change and adapt to new circumstances would quickly deteriorate and die (stimulus–no response). While many of us resist change in some form or another, and while some older people may be more set in their ways, elders do change, often in the form of making adjustments. Rigidity in older people is a stereotype—substitute the word "adjust" for "change." Consider the challenges today's older adults faced in their lifetime, from the Great Depression, World War II, and the Korean War through the increasingly rapid pace of life and change that began in the 1960s. Adjusting to significant change was and continues to be imperative. Accordingly, we suggest throwing out the word "senile" and replace it with "cognitive decline."

> *"What you lose in fast, you gain in savvy."*
> — Old sheriff in *Gunsmoke*

"When more recent memory fails, older adults try to restore balance to their lives by retrieving earlier memories. When eyesight fails, they use the mind's eye to see. When hearing goes, they listen to sounds from the past" (Ronch & Goldfield 2003, p. 106).

Older people don't learn.

None other than Sigmund Freud espoused this myth saying, "Old people are no longer educable." Indeed, until quite recently, most researchers were convinced that the human brain follows a similar pattern of deterioration, believing that brain power peaked at about age 40 and then went predictably downhill. However, recent studies indicate that this turns out to be false. While our physical functioning may decline, the human mind is much more flexible and adaptable. In fact, in *The Synaptic Self*, researcher Joseph E. LeDoux describes the effect of experience on increasing the number of synapses in the brain. When we use it we not only don't lose it, but the brain expands (LeDoux 2002).

Two aspects of learning do decrease as we age (Rowe & Kahn 1998). The speed of processing information diminishes, as well as the ability to do two things at the same time (such as reading and listening to music.) However, the ability to learn complex knowledge and behaviors is unrelated to age (Baltes & Smith 2003). In addition, older people have some reduction in explicit memory, such as a specific name, number, or location. Other kinds of memory show little or no decline, such as working memory, learned routines such as many daily activities like bathing and eating (Rowe & Kahn 1998).

The brain is quite agile and, as we age, different regions start pulling together to make the whole organ work better than the sum of its parts. So, if the left side of the brain begins to deteriorate, such as with a reduction in the ability to use math or the loss of some short-term memory, the right side crosses over to compensate. As we age, the barriers between the hemispheres seem to fall, and the two halves increasingly work together (Kluger 2006).

Dr. Cohen believes, "Clearly, aging presents a great scientific opportunity for exploration, but more important, aging and creativity present an unparalleled opportunity for us as individuals to grow as we grow older in ways that in younger years we could not even have dreamed" (Cohen 2000, p. 66).

At 91, Dale Corson, PhD, President Emeritus, Cornell University reflects on his advancing age. "I've lost my ability to perform mathematics relative to my younger years. But, after I retired in 1979, I spent most of the next 15 years working in

Washington for the National Academy of Sciences, National Academy of Engineers, National Science Foundation, World Bank and the White House."

Older people are unattractive and sexless.

In her 93 years of living, Brenda Euland published six million words, introduced bobbed hair to Greenwich Village and the world, was knighted by the King of Norway, and set an international swimming record for over-80-year-olds. She wrote every day of her life. Here is one of her snippets:

> Sometimes people complain—my children and others—that I dress so unstylishly [sic], so eccentrically, indeed so badly. I say this: If I did not wear torn pants, orthopedic shoes, frantic disheveled hair, that is to say, if I did not tone down my beauty, people would go mad. Married men would run amuck.

While sexual activity may decrease in old age, impacted by cultural norms, health, and the availability of a partner, the basic need for affectionate and physical contact persists throughout life. In their book, *Still Sexy After All These Years? The 9 Unspoken Truths About Women's Desire After 50,* authors Leah Kliger and Deborah Nedelman combined academic research with the art of storytelling to give a comprehensive look at the spectrum of desire and to address the concept of sexual self-esteem in older women across the United States. Notes one interviewee, "It's time to throw out the hogwash and learn the surprising truth about women's sexuality in the last five decades of life." Kliger and Nedelman found that, "Sexual desire changes beyond 50, but not necessarily in the ways you may think. Loss of sexual self-esteem is not an inevitable consequence of growing old!" (http://www.womenbeyond50.com) (Kliger & Nedelman 2006).

It should also be noted that there are many creative ways to express one's sexuality, such as:

- ▌ Touching every hour
- ▌ Leaving a love message each day or relating a sexy story
- ▌ Creating a sexy space
- ▌ Playing with kisses and the like (intercourse is not the only sex that counts).

If, however, couples did not express their sexuality easily as younger adults, it may be difficult to do so in later years.

Four Models of Aging

Social gerontologists address at least four significant aging models, all of which contain factors that must be considered when seeking to age successfully. The first two models—*diminishment* and *leisure*—currently dominate much of Western cultural belief systems, although the second two models—*achievement* and *spiritual growth*—are rapidly gaining in popularity. As they are briefly discussed, keep in mind that "the map is not the territory," that is, a model is only one representation of reality and has its limitations.

The Diminishment Model

This model tends to promote the perception that aging primarily brings a series of problems that must be managed as we experience physical and mental deterioration. Unfortunately, the modern Western medical model of reducing people to biological problems and deficits supports it. According to this model, it is appropriate and expected that people disengage from earlier roles and activities as they age, withdrawing from society. Contrary to these perceptions, while bodily functions obviously do decline with age, the vast majority of people over age 65 remain healthy and active.

However, while true, we can't ignore the fact that not all aging is considered positive. Many people's experiences include arthritis, aching backs, menopause, prostate enlargement, impotence, hair loss, crow's feet, and diminished mobility.

Many elders have more time to volunteer, bestowing blessings on others as well as themselves. President Jimmy and Rosalyn Carter are examples of life expansion, not diminishment. The 1991 Commonwealth Fund Productive Aging Survey depicted the percentages of older persons volunteering at different ages. Even in their early to mid-eighties, more than one-fourth (28%) of older persons were still doing volunteer work (http://www.cmwf.org).

Age	% Volunteering
55–59	31.0%
60–64	26
65–69	27
70–74	26.3
75–79	23.2
80–84	28
85 and older	9.4

On the other hand, it might be argued that there is great value in having less energy; it induces a greater sense of joy in simple things, such as smelling a rose or petting a cat. For thousands of years, Eastern spiritual traditions have extolled the value of slowing down and meditating. There is an element of joy in being dependent upon others. For one thing, it provides professionals with an opportunity to exercise their caregiving skills.

The Leisure Model

Leisure might be defined as engaging in a satisfying activity free from any obligations. People who engage in or dream about pursuing a leisurely lifestyle often speak about traveling, touring the country in a Winnebago, or playing golf at least three times a week. They may adopt a radical consumer mentality, asserting, "I plan to spend it all and leave nothing behind." The challenge involves enjoying one's expanded free time in retirement by keeping "busy," however that plays itself out. Unfortunately, busyness does not always quench the thirst for meaning in one's life, an essential dimension in living a long, healthy life.

Many people struggle to survive and arrive at the day when they can retire. However, the question begs itself: for what purpose? Retirement years are not just for enjoying leisure activities but for harvesting the fruits of our experiences and learning. What lessons have I learned that I can build upon and perhaps pass on to others?

In *Aging Well: Surprising Guideposts To A Happier Life*, George Vaillant, MD, reports on the results of the landmark Harvard Adult Study of Adult Development that was conducted over a period of fifty years by the Harvard Medical School. He outlines four basic activities that make retirement rewarding:

- Replacing work mates with another social network;
- Rediscovering how to play;
- Engaging in some creative enterprises; and
- Continuing life-long learning (Vaillant 2002).

The Achievement Model

Comprehensive research sponsored by HSBC Bank (2005) supports the premise that many people have a new vision of later life as a time of opportunity and reinvention, rather than one of rest and relaxation. The *Future of Retirement* research, commissioned and undertaken between September and October 2004, examines global attitudes and approaches to later life (http://www.hsbc.com/hsbc/retirement_future/2005-research-summary). You *can* teach an old dog new tricks. Grandma Moses didn't start painting until age 75. Giuseppe Verdi wrote his opera *Falstaff* at age 80. George Burns was still entertaining as he was approaching his one-hundredth birthday. Jessica Tandy was in her eighties when she starred in *Driving Miss Daisy*. Sir Winston Churchill was 65 when he became Prime Minister during World War II, later receiving the Nobel Prize in Literature at 79. And we all have known or read of at least one such exemplar of elderly achievement who is not a celebrity. These come to mind:

- Betty Jo Harvey is 71, a mother of five, a long-time registered nurse, and a Red Cross Volunteer for 32 years. Active with the North Central Texas Chapter and with the Red Cross National Headquarters, the National Association of Area Agencies on Aging honored her as a MetLife Foundation *Older Volunteers Enrich America Award* recipient. Among her volunteer roles are traveling on a moment's notice to assist at disaster sites around the country.
- Robert Barnes, MD, now in his eighties, wrote his autobiographical book, *The Good Doctor is Naked: Finding the Human Beneath My Mask*. Professionally successful as a practicing physician, hospital administrator, and medical educator,

he shares his personal journey metaphorically, in which he began well into elderhood of putting on, and then subsequently removing, his "masks" of strength, power, competency, and professionalism. Now a trained spiritual counselor, he describes the process of removing the "MD" mask, which he had assumed in order to hide the shame he felt as a boy of his father's suicide (Barnes 2004).

The widespread assumption that elders don't pull their weight is wrong because the measures are wrong. Many activities are not counted as productive, yet if elders stopped working for pay or as volunteers, the economy, we suspect, would be severely impacted negatively. As one elder said recently, "Where would this country be without us retired people to volunteer? The economy *depends* on us." Elders are more likely to read newspapers, vote, and follow civic and political events.

To be healthy, elders will need to develop a social portfolio [note the model below] as well as a financial portfolio, balancing individual as well as group activities, believes Dr. Cohen, who also views the models of aging differently in his description of the four human potential phases:

- *Midlife Reevaluation Phase*. Occurs between the ages of 40 and 60. Desire to seek and create meaning in life.
- *Liberation Phase*. Sixties to early seventies. Fewer responsibilities and new freedoms. "I've always wanted to . . ." "If not now, when?"
- *Summing-Up Phase*. Seventies or older. Finding the larger meaning in the story of our lives and giving back in the form of wisdom.
- *Encore Phase*. Eighties or older. Making lasting contributions. Taking care of unfinished business (model by Cohen 2000; examples by J. Henry).

The Spiritual Growth Model

Spirituality is not limited to the confines of organized religion, but embraces the sacralization of the self and the world surrounding us. Spirituality embraces the numinous and the mysterious. It is the ability to find the sacred virtually at every point of time and in everything one does, leading to a deep sense of corporate and individual purpose and meaning. Regardless of one's relationship to an organized religion, growing older is a time of deepening spiritual awareness and growth. According to Dr. Richard H. Gentzler, Jr., United Methodist Church Director, Center on Aging and Older Adult Ministries, older adults are looking for specific qualities in a church including:

- A church that helps them deepen their relationship with God;
- A church that provides the freedom for them to seek, doubt, and ask questions related to a growing faith;
- A church that provides opportunities for them to be in relationship with others, including children, youth, and adults of all ages;

- A church where the Word of God is proclaimed with clarity, assurance, and love;
- A church that honestly wrestles with the tough issues of life and death;
- A church that provides older adults with the opportunity to learn and serve;
- A church that values the wisdom, experience, and faith of older adults;
- A church that encourages the faith development of older adults;
- A church that equips older adults for living as faithful Christians;
- A church that is accessible and free of barrier (Gentzler 2005, p. 10).

Unfortunately, a number of churches appear less interested in meeting the needs of elders than in developing programming aimed at younger families, children, and youth.

The Harvard Adult Study highlighted several key dimensions one needs to cultivate to age well, most of which involve the inward journey of deepening:

- A sense of generativity, investing oneself in something that will outlive us;
- A sense of tolerance, patience, open-mindedness, understanding, compassion;
- Maintaining health: abstaining from smoking and alcohol abuse, maintaining a healthy weight, a stable marriage, exercise, having adaptive coping skills;
- A sense of joy in life;
- A sense of subjective life satisfaction not found in outside measurements;
- Instead of viewing the second half as a time of decline, we need a vision of life as a time to discover inner richness and transformation. Out of inner growth comes "sage-ing," where healers and role models for future generations are born (Vaillant 2002).

Four Models

- Diminishment—aging primarily seen as a series of problems that must be managed
- Leisure— engaging in satisfying retirement activities free from any obligation
- Achievement—later life as a time of opportunity and reinvention
- Spiritual Growth—heightened sense of connecting with the sacredness of oneself and the surrounding world

---

If we are truly to transform eldercare, then as a society we must not only examine elderhood in today's world, but be willing to make changes in how we care holistically for an aging population. So, we might tell the Velveteen Rabbit that what is real *can* change. We can keep that which is useful and healthy and create new ways of seeing and caring for the wise ones in our society.

The Worth of Elders:
What Will They Be Good For?

When we first heard about physician Bill Thomas's book, *What Are Old People For?*, instinctively we found ourselves wanting to insert a new word into its title—*What Are Old People* Good *For?* (Thomas 2004). Like so many people in our American culture, we tend to insert this word because of having been programmed throughout a lifetime to believe that old people are hardly good for anything. We live in a culture dominated by the glorification and power of adulthood, whereas elders are generally viewed as being "over-the-hill" people who suffer from physical and mental decline, draining society's resources.

The world of aging portrayed in the mass media has not traditionally been an enjoyable or positive one. The elderly suffer from negative stereotyping on television as much as any other social group.

Even *many* professional caregivers stereotype older people. Dr. Thomas tells the story about giving a speech at the University of Southern California's renown Center of Gerontology. He asked how many in the audience had spoken the word "elderhood" during the past week and only one person raised a hand. In contrast to the word "childhood," "elderhood" is not even in the dictionary.

Being and Doing: Two Intertwining Ways

Founder of the international Eden Alternative™ long-term care movement, Dr. Thomas sharply challenges this stereotypical belief system and envisions a human life cycle that promotes a positive elderhood for all. He expresses this vision essentially in terms of *being* and *doing*. "Humans are interesting creatures," he asserts. "They are able to create an amalgam or blend of the two fundamental energies of *being* and *doing*."

In his book, *The Way of the Physician*, philosopher, historian, and prolific writer Jacob Needleman points out that there are two serpents rather than one in most images of the caduceus, which is widely accepted as the emblem of health care and is applicable to all care providers (Needleman 1985). Like Dr. Thomas, he suggests that the two serpents essentially represent two fundamental energies of *doing* and *being*. More left brain than right brain, one of these two energies focuses more upon rational, analytical, technical exploration and competence. It serves primarily as the *doing* aspect of health care. Its complementary opposite force concentrates most of its attention upon *being*; it is relational and concerned with compassionate caring. Both of these energies apply equally to health care and healing; one without the other leaves the health care and healing system crippled, and to some extent, the caregivers and healers—and their clients and patients—are likewise compromised.

These two energies can be viewed as flowing from archetypes, a word adapted by the Swiss psychologist Carl Jung to convey deeply rooted and innate elements of human consciousness that can erupt upon our awareness from time to time from the unconscious, often as imagery or other symbolic forms. Archetypes are not static principles but life forces in the psyche from centuries of life experiences.

Humans come into this world with a cognitive apparatus somewhat like the hard drive of a computer, already formatted and programmed to interact with certain things in certain ways. For example, a newborn baby knows instinctively what to do with a mother in terms of feeding; the archetype of mother is embedded in the child in terms of both biological and psychological instincts.

In contemporary holistic health care practice, *being* and *doing* can provide a framework for the underlying therapies as well as descriptors of the two poles of any approach to health and wellness that is based in achieving some optimal balance. For instance, holistic nursing therapies are usefully so grouped: "Doing therapies include almost all forms of modern medicine, such as medications, procedures, dietary manipulations, radiation, and acupuncture. In contrast, being therapies do not employ things, but instead use states of consciousness . . . imagery, prayer, meditation, and quiet contemplation, as well as the presence and intention of the nurse. These techniques are therapeutic because of the power of the psyche to affect the body" (Dossey, Keegan, & Guzzetta 2005, pp. 12–16).

In general terms, the energies of *doing* and *being* surface within the Chinese symbols of yang and yin, which in turn find useful therapeutic expression in many aspects of traditional Chinese medicine. They can also represent the masculine *doing* and feminine *being* that reside in both men and women, although generally the masculine finds dominant expression in men and the feminine in women. The two energies come together in the form of the active sperm and the receptive egg to conceive a new life.

Another perspective on interdependent distinction of *doing* and *being* emerges from two functions of sight. In order for us to see, the eye must synchronize focused and peripheral vision. When we view an object, we experience both focused content (doing) and diffused context and background (being). Without both aspects, we simply could not see anything.

Characteristics of Being and Doing

To further understanding and appreciate these fundamental energies, we suggest breaking them down into five characteristics and their opposites (Henry & Henry 1999). Again, we are reminded that these dynamic energies embody themselves in both men and women, although, as we shall see, they find dominant expression in different stages of the life cycle in different cultures.

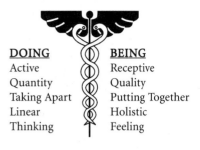

DOING	BEING
Active	Receptive
Quantity	Quality
Taking Apart	Putting Together
Linear	Holistic
Thinking	Feeling

Active versus Receptive

Doing is active. Activity happens when we come into a relationship with the visible, tangible, material world and we seek to change or alter that world in some manner. We actively attend to our chores, to our homework, and to our jobs. The fruit of activity includes productivity, efficiency, and achievement. Activity comes easily for most of us because it is so practical and applicable to everyday living. We find it easy and straightforward to count the number of things we do or to check them off on a list.

In contrast to the activity of *doing*, *being* is receptive. Like the egg, it represents an openness and responsiveness to impending events and information. It stands willing to receive and nurture that which is given. Receptivity involves bringing one's quiet attention to self and to relationships with others, nature, and the sacred. The receptive person does not attempt to force experience but is willing to allow it to simply happen. Jungian analyst Irene Claremont de Castillego underlines that the deepest communication takes place in moments of silence (Castillego 1973).

Obviously, receptivity is a key skill vital to effective intervention. To practice effectively, the healthcare professional must be receptive to the information and complaints of the patient. Research and investigative endeavors must seek to suspend preconceived assumptions and be receptive to new information.

Quantity versus Quality

The next two sets of opposites can engender considerable controversy in health care. Quantity refers to the concern for the amount, size, or body of something. Because of financial concerns, staff limitations, and other pressures, many managers and professionals often find themselves driven to assembly line, time-pressured health care. Without an appropriate centering of attention upon quantity and production, upon output and outcomes, quotas and profit, many organizations will simply cease to exist. However, an obsession with quantifiable short-term results can devastate human caring in health care.

Quality refers to doing the right things and doing things right. It displays a rich interest in excellence and worth. Obviously, few, if any people, would be attracted to a healthcare practitioner or institution known for inferior service.

Quality also embodies such attributes as unconditional positive regard, understanding, honesty, and empathy. In health care, as well as through clinical competence, the quality of a relationship with a patient can be heard in the gentle tone of voice and seen in a loving touch and in the connection through the eyes. The phrase "relationship-centered care" captures the essence of quality attention.

Taking Apart Versus Putting Together

Another characteristic of doing involves the dynamic of taking apart. In a very micro sense, the healthcare professional is continuously taking apart, dissecting nature and the human body, examining individual components of a system. "Taking apart" something serves us well in terms of problem solving and getting past vague generalizations such as "We've got a morale problem."

Putting together operates as a feminine *being* alternative. It has to do with understanding the interconnectedness of people, data, and objects. For the surgeon, it means putting back together that which was taken apart. For a medical technician, it involves understanding the interrelationship of biological systems with other structures. In terms of management, it encompasses a participatory style of operating, emphasizing team building and seeking consensus.

Linear Versus Holistic

Doing energy tends to operate in a *linear* fashion. It utilizes step-by-step sequential thinking, as would be involved in a serial operating procedure. Concern focuses upon the length of something or the length of time required to complete a task. Linear thinking tends to be one-dimensional and becomes especially important when fitting together elaborate elements of significant complexity.

The opposite of linear is a holistic, multidimensional approach. It is seeing the whole as greater than the sum of its parts. It emphasizes systems interrelationships and harmony, seeing the impact of one part or decision upon the whole. At the individual level, it involves understanding and acting upon the premise that one *always does* make a difference, however small, in the overall scheme of things. A holistic practitioner seeks to become a channel through which flow healing energies.

Thinking versus Feeling

Finally, *doing* energy emphasizes the importance of thinking processes. It utilizes logical analysis, the use of intellect, and critical judgment. The thinking function dominates Western culture, focusing upon the head in contrast to the heart. Rene Descartes' "I think, therefore I am" serves as the mantra of this orientation, as does Hamlet's, "Nothing is good or bad, but thinking makes it so."

Feeling obviously involves the expression of emotion and sentiment. However, feeling resonates with broader qualities. Feeling also has to do with making decisions based upon their impact on others. A feeling orientation values people and acts in their best interest. The expressions of feeling in health care are not dispensable but vital to whole-person care.

Those with a more hard-nosed, bottom-line, common-sense style of thinking in health care and business may reject the above descriptions as too subjective, theoretical, and a waste of time. Such judgments mirror the current, overwhelmingly *doing*, masculine nature of many organizations. However, undervaluing the feminine *being* is like cutting off one leg. *Doing* energies unbalanced by the *being* energies often result in an unbalanced orientation toward productivity, efficiency, and control. By most enlightened management standards, nit picking, tunnel vision, and obsession with short-term results deteriorate customer relations and profitability over the long haul.

Susan Lucia Annunzio, Chairman and CEO of the Hudson Highland Center For High Performance, and her team completed world-wide research to identify the factors that accelerate or inhibit high performance in work groups. As reported in her book, *Contagious Success: Spreading High Performance Throughout Your Organization*, their research found three factors that distinguished high-performing workgroups:

▌ Valuing people
▌ Optimizing critical thinking
▌ Seizing opportunities

According to their study, there is quantifiable proof of a direct correlation between how employers treat people and financial results, and this supports other studies that link employee attitudes and behaviors, customer satisfaction, and profitability. The team found that the single biggest impediment to high performance world-wide is short-term thinking. "To meet quarterly financial goals, companies are trying to do more with less, overworking their people, and cutting muscle along with the fat. Regrettably, they may be sacrificing long-term sustainability for short-term results" (Annunzio 2004, p. 17).

Elders as Masters of Balance: Being and Doing United

An ever-expanding body of research is being conducted contributing to the perspective that as we age, we bring *doing* and *being* into greater balance. More than ever before, health promotion therapies, nutrition, exercise, and general wellness activities make it possible for elders to remain active and productive well into their seventies and eighties. In varying ways, pensions, savings accounts, Medicare, and Social Security allow many elders to pursue purposeful and satisfying work activities, for pay or as volunteers.

At the same time, evidence continues to expand testifying to the reality that, as they age, many elders become masters of *being,* raising it up as a vital part of daily life for all ages. In this respect, as more and more boomers enter elderhood, their contribution to the well-being of society and to the environment will continue to expand.

Eden Alternative™: A Transformational Approach to Eldercare

We already mentioned Bill Thomas, MD, founder of the Eden Alternative™ movement and a geriatrician with an international reputation in his field. This long-term care movement has its roots in a 1991 pilot project initiated by Dr. Thomas and seeded with a grant from the state of New York. According to Thomas, it is more than just fuzzy props, potted plants, animals, and the presence of children. The Eden philosophy is summed up in this poster hanging on the wall at St. John's Retirement Community, a registered Eden home: "*Our elders do not live in our facility. We work in their home.*"

Being concerns itself with things that cannot be seen. In an Eden facility, this has to do with creating and nurturing relationships based upon trust, respect, optimism, and mutual caring. In an Eden home, *being* surfaces as the opposite of dictated efficiency, rules, and conformity. Residents determine when and how long to sleep, when and what to eat, and when and in what to participate.

It's about giving people a reason to live, an approach that also impacts the bottom line. For extensive data related to such issues as staff turnover and absenteeism, facility cost reduction, infection rates, reduced medication usage and use of patient restraints, visit http://edenalt.com/data.htm.

Bill explains how his work as a physician evolved in this direction. "After beginning my work in a nursing home, it quickly became obvious that just prescribing drugs was not going to cut it for these people. I witnessed the slow, agonizing death of good people who suffered from an emptiness of spirit. They felt they had no reason to live. The problem wasn't about sufficient medical treatment, but about fulfillment in life. Nursing homes have long tended to confuse fulfillment with busyness. So, we began to experiment with alternative approaches, infusing the environment with huge numbers of plants, animals, and children. It included a radically, redefined relationship between management and staff. The goal was to create an environment that was warm, suffused with life, laughter and song in a natural, everyday manner, but not as an organized, structured activity" (Henry & Henry 2002, pp. 183–84). For a more in-depth description of an Eden facility in this book, see Suellen Beatty, "Living Life in the Garden of Eden: Sherbrooke Community Centre," in Section 3.

Today, the Eden philosophy is being embraced all over the world with more than 400 affiliated facilities implementing the philosophy. Bill regards it as a social movement. He believes that the world can be made a better place by innovatively caring for frail elders. If this can be accomplished, it offers important lessons for society in general. In reality, the way we care for our elders mirrors the health of our culture. He reports, "One of the most important things elders have to teach us is about how to create a truly human society. A society caring for frail, elderly people in a tender and compassionate way is a better society in general. If we keep our promise to them, we actually make a better life for ourselves" (Henry & Henry 2002, p. 184).

Gerotranscendence: A Transformational Philosophy of Aging

A word coined by gerontologist Lars Tornstam, PhD, gerotranscendence means elders rising above the cultural demands of adulthood and moving in the direction of maturation, wisdom, and spiritual growth. Dr. Tornstam currently holds the first Swedish chair in social gerontology at Uppsala University in Sweden. The concept of gerotranscendence was based upon qualitative and quantitative research from 1990 through 2001 involving interviews and surveys with thousands of men and women ages 65 to 104 (Tornstam 2005). He asserts that many of our attitudes about elders emerge from Western culture and white middle-class adult hopes for successful aging with its emphasis upon *doing*, productivity, efficiency, individuality, independence, competition, and the desire to accumulate wealth. To the extent that it fails to live up to these standards, old age becomes a burdensome time of diminishment and misery. While this is true of some elders and especially of those who succumb to such stereotypical assumptions, Tornstam's research exposes these "facts" as essentially false, in light of a natural progression toward holistic maturation. While this seed of maturation and the energy to germinate it exists in every human being, many older people find these impossible cultural norms difficult to overcome and therefore tend to develop anger, depression, and disgust with themselves, believing that life in old age is a waste.

Both Thomas and Tornstam call upon elders to resist this projection of adulthood into senior years and to embrace the energy of *being*, with its power to ignite a sense of fulfillment and purpose as they age. These elders find themselves able to transcend the competitive juices of middle age and enter a time of mutuality, cooperation, spiritual growth, depth of wisdom, and the promotion of peace.

The Worth of Elders:
What *Are* They Good For?

Contrary to common Western cultural norms that have influenced us for many decades, elders are good for a great number of things. We choose to highlight just a few of their more critical contributions as they surface from the energy and attributes of *being*. Most of the following characteristics flow from Tornstam's research on gerotranscendence.

- Teachers of receptivity
- Pursuers of quality
- Integrators and makers of connections
- Embracers of holism
- Relaters with feeing

Teachers of Receptivity

This attribute of mature elderhood often emanates from a life review process and results in a general sense of self-acceptance. An elder looks through an imaginary rearview mirror, identifying and reflecting upon the high points and low times. The various aspects of one's overall personality are brought to consciousness, as well as what Carl Jung called the *shadow*: that part of one's own individual consciousness that has been kept packed away and out of sight due to its self-perceived fearfulness. (Poet Robert Bly aptly termed the human shadow as "the long bag we drag behind us.") One learns to accept achievements and failures, finding value in all of them. It includes being receptive to one's physical situation and its limitations.

Receptivity also surfaces in the form of enjoying solitude, finding peace and satisfaction in the "ground of being," a term coined by Paul Tillich, one of the twentieth century's most prominent theologians. In addition, these elders often are more other-directed in terms of displaying a profound interest in environmental surroundings, people, nature, and the like.

A nursing home resident said, "Lack of physical strength keeps me inactive and often silent. They call me senile, but senility is just a convenient peg on which to hang non-conformity" (Dass 2000, p. 38). As we age, "attention—curiosity, openness of heart ands mind, sensitivity to the souls of others, and a capacity to wait—may better suit the season" (Raines 1998, p. 105).

Pursuers of Quality

This dimension of gerotranscendence involves putting first things first—enjoying basic life activities such as rest, walking, dining, and relating to the external world. It includes expressing gratitude for simple pleasures.

The number of overall relationships may begin to decline as people age, perhaps because of reduced mobility and/or sensing that the end of one's life is drawing nearer. Yet interactions tend to have more depth and intimacy. *Quality* takes precedence over the quantity of relationships, one reason why many eldercare service providers inform us that no matter how much they put into their work, elderly clients give back a thousandfold.

This aspect also includes quality of work. In the most complete sense of the word, all people work. However, for many elders who are freer from financial and time constraints, work takes place for the sake of one's soul. There is a deepening sense of being "called" to perform a task. For instance, a 70-year-old friend of ours built a carpentry shop in his backyard and makes beautiful wooden, painted ducks that sell for a considerable amount of money. His creative work reflects an element of mastery rather than production and a high degree of self-fulfillment as opposed to drudgery.

Integrators and Makers of Connections

Elders reaching this level of maturation aging enjoy synthesizing, seeing the connections between people and things. They tend to be less judgmental and more open to diversity and paradox, as well as appreciating the truths of various traditions and viewpoints. They enjoy seeing linkages to earlier generations and seem especially able to relate to grandchildren.

Bridge building is valued, which contributes to a talent of peacemaking. Bill Thomas addresses this feature in terms of three dimensions: Making peace with oneself, with one's family, and in the world.

Dr. Cohen suggests that when elders tell their story, they combine qualities of creativity and aging to become "the keepers of the culture, the long recognized role of elders, passing on values, wisdom, and a way of life, whether in the culture of a family, a geographic community, or a people bound by ideology" (Cohen 2000, p. 234).

Embracers of Holism

This aspect of gerotranscendence includes a sense of cosmic communion, believing that everything is interrelated and connected to the whole. There evolves a growing sense that one's life has a purpose, that one is living a legacy and leaving it for future generations to appreciate.

A redefinition of time occurs, with an emphasis upon its circular nature as opposed to linear time, as postulated by numerous cultures throughout the ages, by cosmologists and quantum theorists, from Einstein onwards, and by contemporary thinkers on human health and development. Rabbi Zalman Schachter-Shalomi, in the context of his "sage-ing" and "spiritual aging" approach perspective, has noted, "Time is stretchable, not linear, so we can reframe and reshape it using contemplative techniques" (Schachter-Shalomi 1995, p. 93). Time seems to move both more rapidly and slowly, perhaps especially for elders, more rapidly when engaged in a satisfying experience and more slowly in the midst of stress or pain. In his pioneering work, *Space, Time, and Medicine*, Larry Dossey, MD, expands upon such experiences of time (Dossey 1982).

We find ourselves enthralled by expressions of wisdom from these elders. Returning to the caduceus, we described the energy of *doing* as flowing from the masculine archetype and the energy of *being* as emerging from feminine essence. Sophia is the personification of feminine energy and is known as the goddess of wisdom. Accordingly, because of their many life experiences, elders are givers of wisdom, purposely applying knowledge and experience with common sense and insight.

Somewhat related, there is a decreased fear of death. "Every spiritual tradition [believes] that preparation for death is the single most important spiritual practice available to us through our lives" (Dass 2000, p. 150). Death is absolutely vital to making life meaningful; for example, nearing-death experiences may include the qualities of relaxation, withdrawal, radiance, silence, and the sacred (Singh 2000).

Relaters with Feeling

With respect to this attribute, Laura Carstensen and her team at Stanford University researched the emotional states of people from ages 18 to 94 years and concluded that elders are more emotionally astute and balanced (Carstensen et al. 2000). The emotional system "works" well even in very old age; the ability to experience emotions deeply and regulate them effectively may even improve with age. Because of years of experience, elders seem to know what kinds of events increase or decrease emotions and therefore are better able to attain balance by minimizing negative emotions and maximizing positive ones.

Once more, it is vital to note that while the seed of growth toward maturity and gerotranscendence exists in all people, it may never germinate for some because of social, psychological, and environmental dynamics. Grumpy, stubborn, narrow-minded, and decrepit, some limp their way to death's door. Others display flickers of growth and, if observed over a longer period of time, they show flashes of the attributes of holistic aging, although sometimes these behaviors are judged as signs of pathology, dementia, or drug use (Tornstam 2005).

In his superb book, *America the Wise*, subtitled *The Longevity Revolution and the True Wealth of Nations*, Theodore Roszak trumpets the need to promote elder values in our society and speaks optimistically about the overall cultural impact of aging baby boomers. He foresees elders having greater involvement in the community, with their making substantial personal contributions in terms of time and energy to social issues (Roszak 1998). As baby boomers push into their sixties and seventies, we can expect the seeds of gerotranscendence to germinate throughout U.S. society (Tornstam 2005).

The challenge for those who provide services to elders requires helping people (including caregivers themselves) to adopt more healthy perceptions of the aging process and to explore and implement innovative eldercare models, strategies, and resources. The challenge involves turning flickers and flashes into bonfires. In this respect, two of the more innovative organizations are Second Journey (www.secondjourney.org) and Pioneer Network (www.pioneernetwork.net). Hopefully, the remainder of this book will serve as a guide in this respect.

References

Annunzio, S. with S. McGowan. 2004. *Contagious Success: Spreading High Performance Throughout Your Organization*. New York: Penguin.

AORN Journal. 2002. http://www.surgery.org.

Baltes, P.B., & J. Smith. 2003. New frontiers in the future of aging: From successful aging of the young old to the dilemmas of the Fourth Age. *Gerontology: Behavioural Science Section/Review* 49:123–35.

Barnes, R. 2004. *The Good Doctor is Naked: Finding the Human Beneath My Mask*. Lincoln, NE: iUniverse.

Butler, R. 1969. Age-ism: Another form of bigotry. *The Gerontologist* 9:243–46.

Carstensen, L., M. Pasupathi, U. Mayr, & J. Nesselroade. 2000. Emotional experiences in everyday life across the adult life span. *Journal of Personality and Social Psychology* 79(4):644–55.

Castillego, I. 1973. *Knowing Woman: A Feminine Psychology*. New York: Harper & Row.

Cohen, G. 2000. *The Creative Age: Awakening Human Potential in the Second Half of Life*. New York: Avon Books.

Dass, R. 2000. *Still Here: Embracing Aging, Changing and Dying*. New York: Riverside Books.

Dossey, B.M., L. Keegan, and C.E. Guzzetta. 2005. *Holistic Nursing: A Handbook for Practice*. 4th ed. Sudbury, MA: Jones and Bartlett, pp. 12–16.

Dossey, L. 1982. *Space, Time, and Medicine*. Boston: Shambhala.

Dychtwald, K. 1999. *Age Power: How the 21st Century Will Be Ruled by the New Old*. NY: Archer Putnam.

Feder, Judith. July-August 2005. "Do older Americans hide assets to qualify for Medicaid?" *Aging Today*, p. 9.

Gentzler, R. Fall, 2005. "What do seniors want in a church?" *Center Sage* (newsletter). Nashville, TN: Center on Aging and Older-Adult Ministries.

Harkness, H. 1999. *Don't Stop the Career Clock*. Palo Alto, CA: Davies-Black.

Henry, L. & J. Henry. 1999. *Reclaiming Soul in Health Care*. Chicago: AHA Press.

Henry, L. & J. Henry. 2002. *The Soul of the Physician*. Chicago: AMA Press.

Hooyman, N. & H. Kiyak. 2004. *Social Gerontology*. Boston: Allyn and Bacon.

Kliger, L. & D. Nedelman. 2006. *Still Sexy After All These Years? The 9 Unspoken Truths About Women's Desire After 50*. New York: Perigee/Penguin.

Kluger, J. January 16, 2006. "The Surprising Power of the Aging Brain." *Time Magazine* 167(3).

LeDoux, J.E. 2002. *The Synaptic Self*. New York: Viking Penguin.

Needleman, J. 1985. *The Way of the Physician*. San Francisco: Harper & Row.

Raines, R. 1998. *A Time to Live: Seven Steps of Creative Aging*. NY: Plume Printing.

Ronch, J. & J. Goldfield. 2003. *Mental Wellness in Aging: Strength-Based Approaches*. Baltimore: Health Professions Press.

Roszak, T. 1998. *America The Wise: The Longevity Revolution and the True Wealth of Nations*. New York: Houghton Mifflin.

Rowe, J and R. Kahn. 1998. *Successful Aging*. NY: Dell Publishing.

Sauer, R. Fall, 2005. "Senior adult spirituality group." *Center Sage* (newsletter). Nashville, TN: Center on Aging and Older-Adult Ministries.

Schachter-Shalomi, Z. 1995. *From Age-ing to Sage-ing: A Profound New Vision of Growing Older*. New York: Warner Books.

Singh, K. 2000. *The Grace in Dying: A Message of Hope, Comfort, and Spiritual Transformation*. New York: HarperCollins.

Sloane, T. July 25, 2005. "Opinions-Editorials." *Modern Healthcare*, p. 18.

Thomas, W. 2004. *What Are Old People For?* Acton, MA: VanderWyk & Burnham.

Tornstam, L. 2005. *Gerotranscendence*. New York: Springer Publishing Company.

U.S. Bureau of Statistics. 2000. U.S. Census Bureau Fact Finder. http://factfinder.census.gov.

Vaillant, G. 2002. *Aging Well: Surprising Guideposts to a Happier Life*. Boston: Little, Brown.

Williams, M. 1922. *The Velveteen Rabbit, Or How Toys Become Real*. Various illustrated editions. The original edition, with illustrations by William Nicholson, is available online at either (in zipped form) http://www.gutenberg.org/etext/11757, or http://digital.library.upenn.edu/women/williams/rabbit/rabbit.html.

Section 2
Emerging Innovative Caring Concepts

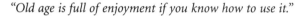

"Old age is full of enjoyment if you know how to use it."

—Seneca
(4 B.C.–65 A.D.)

In This Section . . . Highlights include the first geriatric emergency medicine fellowship, the Hospital Elder Life Program (HELP), and several other inpatient eldercare programs designed to increase beneficial outcomes. Transitional programs to help bridge the gap between the diagnosis of a terminal illness and hospice and additional specific, more holistic caring practices are identified.

BUILDING A NEW GERIATRIC EMERGENCY MEDICINE SUBSPECIALTY

Neal Flomenbaum, MD, FACP, FACEP, and Michael Stern, MD

Issues related to aging are interesting and complex, suggests Neal Flomenbaum, MD, Emergency Physician-in-Chief at New York-Presbyterian Hospital, Weill Cornell Medical Center, who heads a new, first-of-its-kind geriatric emergency medicine fellowship. "When we say someone is old, what do we mean?" Neal asks. "Whenever you use the words 'elderly', 'geriatrics', 'senior citizen,' or any of the current euphemisms or substitute words, you almost always see a frown on someone's face.

"One of the first questions I get when I bring up the subject of geriatric emergency medicine to hospital administrators and clinicians is, 'Who exactly are you talking about?' I know that the reason they ask that question is because they are wondering whether they themselves meet or are close to meeting the definition. Typically, people don't become CEOs, COOs, presidents, deans, or directors of large, prominent organizations until they are at a decent age, and so when I answer that the group I am focusing on is upwards of 75, there is usually a sigh of relief. Perhaps we should start referring to the elderly as 'experienced adults.'"

Neal also is the Medical Director of New York Presbyterian's Emergency Medical Service of over 50 ambulances and a Professor of Clinical Medicine at Weill Medical College of Cornell University. For more than a quarter of a century, he has been involved with efforts to establish and support emergency medicine (EM) as a specialty and to provide the highest-quality EM education and training. He believes that the dynamics of an aging population are rapidly changing and that in the future there will be many more older people functioning well and enjoying life who are living at home or in assisted living facilities. The impetus for developing a new subspecialty in geriatric emergency medicine was spurred by Neal's experiences with an ever-increasing, highly functional geriatric population needing the services provided by emergency departments.

"At New York Presbyterian we do rounds every evening at 7:30 p.m. By that time of night, when there is any degree of overcrowding or when there are fewer total beds available in the hospital than are needed, things tend to back up in the ED [Emergency Department]. Even on good days, the largest ED patient population is usually present during the evening hours. Each evening when I review the active patients shown on our tracking system, I am struck by the number of patients who are in their nineties and one hundreds and who require care for acute problems. Although some come from nursing homes, most come from their own homes, frequently accompanied by spouses and children. I think that this is an important phenomenon. As recently as 10 or 20 years ago, we rarely saw ED patients in their nineties, let alone one hundreds, but it's not unusual anymore. All of the demographics suggest that the segment of the population over age 65 is increasing and is probably increasing more rapidly than any other age group that uses emergency services. Clearly, many people in a variety of disciplines should start thinking about addressing the needs of the elderly."

Neal emphasizes the importance of both fast and accurate diagnosis and treatment of older patients who come to the Emergency Department with acute illnesses or injuries. "If we succeed in rapidly diagnosing and treating their problems, they are more likely to return home and resume their independent lives," he affirms. "Conversely, failing to do so may mean a permanent loss of independence for the patient."

Even though the focus of the geriatric emergency medicine fellowship is on elders 75 and above, patients over 65 currently represent more than 20% of all patients treated in emergency departments, according to Neal. He suggests that age 65 today is equivalent to age 40 about 30–40 years ago and that most people no longer consider 65 years as "old." After age 70 to 75, however, according to Neal, there are significant physiologic changes that will affect everyone to some extent. "Chronological age should not be the major criterion in how we view elders," he explains. "I like to use the analogy of a vintage car; we all know of older cars that have been well cared for, are attractive, and still run fine. On the other hand, there are newer cars that have been neglected and, as a result, don't run well at all. I think that how people age is a combination of lifestyle, how they have maintained their health, and their genetics. These factors are often more important than whether someone is 73 or 83," he states.

The geriatric emergency medicine program will benefit elders in a number of ways, according to Neal. "*All* properly trained emergency physicians are well qualified to deal with geriatric emergencies. They recognize that people at the extremes of age—the very old as well as neonates and infants—often present with significant illnesses, but do not necessarily show signs and symptoms consistent with the seriousness of that illness. The value of creating a subspecialty in geriatric emergency medicine lies in being able to acquire the means to do the kind of clinical and bench research on drug actions, drug interactions, and different therapeutic modalities for the different problems of aging that will have the greatest impact on managing emergencies and providing effective care."

In addition, an organized geriatric emergency medicine subspecialty can involve other members of the health team with ED patients in different ways than they have been involved until now, Neal explains. "One example is to rethink the nature and the extent of the involvement of social services in the ED. Typically, only after we admit patients from the ED to different inpatient services is a social worker's assistance requested for help with the discharge planning and after-hospitalization care. Waiting this long may prolong the patient's length of stay in the hospital, tie up in-patient beds longer, and ultimately turn the Emergency Department into a holding unit for new patients waiting for those beds to become available."

Instead, Neal would like to see a means of providing "discharge planning" for an elderly person who comes to the ED with an acute problem and to use that visit as a barometer of how the individual is doing and what his or her needs may be, in order to prevent a more serious problem from developing. "The signal from the patient might be, 'I'm doing okay; I'm declining gradually, but something just happened this morning and now I'm declining a lot faster. Can you help me? Can you get me back up on that graceful aging curve?' If you could approach someone who gets into trouble that way and not just fix the acute medical or surgical problem, which may be the easy part of it, but figure out why they got into trouble and how to prevent it from happening again, you could turn that ED episode into a bump in the road instead of the *end* of the road.

"Too often we use all of our considerable diagnostic tools to exclude a serious condition such as a fracture and then treat the bruise while never asking the additional questions that we should: We determine that there has been a fall. Although we may even learn that it was a fall getting up from the toilet, we often don't ask the next questions about what may have contributed to the fall or what could have been done to prevent it. If the patient stumbled getting up from the toilet and we know that there is no grab bar next to it, we could show the patient what a grab bar looks like on a computer screen and have the social worker help make arrangements to have one installed the next day, all while the patient is still in the ED! The ED visit should serve as a way of alerting care providers that the patient's environment needs to be evaluated for potential dangers. The emergency visit would then become an opportunity to marry acute care with preventive care. Of course, in order to do this without further adding to the delays in throughput that already paralyze many EDs today, we would have to insure that social workers are always immediately available and also, perhaps, that there is a separate area in the ED to conduct such exchanges."

Because aging individuals are more diverse and complicated physically and emotionally, Neal underscores the importance of care providers understanding these complexities. First, he believes that care providers in general need to know how the aging process affects an individual's ability to respond to acute medical and physical changes. Explains Neal, the degree of aging may not be apparent day to day, but when elderly people experience acute medical or surgical problems, their ability to respond the way we have come to expect may be dramatically different because of their diminished physical reserves.

Neal shares an example of an 83-year-old woman who had complained of not feeling well for a few weeks because of abdominal pains not unlike pains she had experienced in the past. "She was constipated with intermittent pain and had a loss of appetite. A week before we saw her, she had been examined by a gastroenterologist who did not feel that her condition was serious enough to warrant any radiologic studies. She said that she had been told that she was having irregularity and then was given a prescription for a laxative. For a short time she seemed to do somewhat better. But a week later she and her family were concerned that she was just 'not right.' They called and asked if her condition merited an evaluation in the ED. Fortunately, we told her that there was no way to exclude a serious condition without actually examining her and then helped arrange her trip to the ED. Upon arrival, the physical exam revealed nothing very remarkable, but a requested abdominal CT scan surprisingly revealed about 250 ml. of pus in her abdomen. Any patient half her age would probably have had board-like abdominal rigidity characteristic of a perforated viscus, an obvious potentially life-threatening condition. Sometimes you have to appreciate what you don't know. It's a very tricky age group to deal with."

Second, Neal suggests more age-based diagnostic strategies that combine the art and science of medicine with the skills of physicians to diagnose more complex problems. "We need to develop strategies that might not otherwise be used to diagnose similar problems in younger patients." Referring again to the example of the 83-year-old woman, he says, "Somebody younger with the same lack of symptoms probably would not have required a CT scan. However, when people of advanced age present with minimal symptoms, you need to perform diagnostic tests you might not otherwise do, which brings up the question of resources. How are we going to decide who really needs the additional diagnostic studies in that age group? Right now it's an art. Hopefully, in five or ten years we'll know better what the real criteria are or should be and it will be more of a science. For now and for the foreseeable future, any bedside noninvasive means of getting information is particularly valuable. Perhaps a sonogram is indicated because it's noninvasive and can be done quickly and easily at the bedside."

Issues involving healthcare reimbursement for aging individuals are of enormous concern, reports Neal. "Typically, reimbursement for preventive care is less available for elders than is reimbursement for the aftermath of a serious or catastrophic illness requiring hospitalization followed by rehabilitation or long-term care in a nursing home." He suggests the need for economic models to evaluate costs of care. "While there are some economic models currently available, they need to be reexamined and better adjusted for the increasing number of people in that age group, as well as to reflect the changing nature of their condition and overall health and the recent changes in medicine. Over the past 10 years, almost everything medically and surgically has changed, and that will continue to be the case.

"We probably need to enlist the aid of a group of talented economists who can look at people over the age of 80 and then help us develop functional criteria for addressing and anticipating the needs of the elderly in a cost-effective way. Many elders who live at home may have diabetes, hypertension, or other serious, chronic illnesses. We need to look for simple cost-effective screening tests that can be used to diagnose or predict illnesses and help us tailor treatment for these individuals. Hopefully, we can demonstrate afterwards that by providing preventive care earlier, we can help people stay in their homes longer. Compared to the cost of a nursing home, we could potentially save tens or hundreds of thousands of dollars per person."

The initial years of the first two geriatric emergency medicine fellowships were funded by a private donor for one fellow per year. Neal acknowledges that additional resources will be needed before the current funding runs out. "I am hopeful that the data that we are able to gather during this initial period will show the differences that physicians trained in geriatric emergency medicine can make and, as a result, help sustain additional fellowships."

Finally, Neal believes that training physicians in geriatric emergency medicine makes so much sense because older patients frequently experience several different types of medical problems simultaneously, perhaps diabetes or heart disease accompanied by skin lesions or fractures.

"One of the interesting things about emergency medicine," says Michael Stern, MD, the first Geriatric Emergency Medicine Fellow, "is that we are often the front line, acting as the portal into the hospital system. Many times we see people with new complaints and illnesses as they present to a doctor for the first time, so we need to think and act both diagnostically and therapeutically for virtually every single entity that we might encounter. With the older patient population, we must be particularly cognizant of how complex their problems can be.

"Older patients have very different medical issues," explains Michael. "There are geriatric emergency syndromes that we see that are fairly unique to geriatric patients. These patients can present some of the most challenging diagnostic and management dilemmas and, in turn, are often extremely rewarding patients to care for. What we read about in textbooks in terms of how patients classically present with various clinical syndromes or disease states does not apply as readily to older patients. And that's the challenge. They are atypical in their presentations and can present to an ED much later, or their physical exam findings are more subtle. Often, there are multiple complaints that one must sift through in order to discover the central issue that is causing the problem.

"One of the clinical entities that we frequently see in older patients is delirium. There are a number of possible causes, and part of our job is to determine what is causing the mental status changes. Often, what we do or don't do in the Emergency Department can profoundly impact these older patients in terms of both their morbidity and mortality. As a result of the care we provide in the ED, we have the opportunity to help the elderly person overcome a potentially catastrophic illness or event and enable them to go on leading highly functioning lives as independent individuals out in the community. Being aware of all these complex issues is one of the things I find intriguing about emergency medicine and geriatrics coming together."

As the first fellow in an integrated Geriatric Emergency Medicine Fellowship, Michael believes he has an opportunity to advance the new subspecialty. "It's my belief that with continued learning, teaching, and clinical research, I'll help [achieve] that goal. Geriatric emergency medicine makes perfect sense because of the demographics of the older population and what emergency medicine is all about."

Other syndromes often seen in an ED, according to Michael, include dizziness, hip fractures, depression, anxiety, incontinence, pressure ulcers, and adverse drug reactions often masquerading as other problems as the result of separate undiagnosed or untreated conditions. "The toxicological syndrome of polypharmacy is a huge issue," he states. "Many of the patients in their eighties or nineties who are basically in good health have a number of chronic medical conditions that are well managed, but that require a number of medicines. Although these medicines may work well, at times they can cause side effects or powerful synergies through their interactions. And sometimes, older patients may be taking numerous medicines prescribed by sub-specialists, but they do not have overall management of their medication and general health by a primary care doctor. This can lead to myriad clinical problems, many of which we see in the ED," he cautions.

Michael's fellowship year includes rotations in the ED, rounding with the geriatric service on their inpatient teams, and rounding in the intensive care units. "Some of what we do in the ED impacts the care people get as an inpatient. It's nice to have an interface between what happens on the inpatient service and what happens in the ED because the two are definitely linked. I am learning from them and hopefully will teach them as well. I want to take this information back to the ED to incorporate into both patient care and the education of residents and medical students who are training in the ED."

He also spends time at the Hebrew Home for the Aged (HHAR) in Riverdale, NY, which has a first-of-its-kind inpatient elder abuse unit. "Unfortunately," says Michael, "abuse and neglect cross all socioeconomic lines, and cases are increasing in numbers. We need to be much more vigilant in the ED by recognizing it more readily. It occurs with more frequency than many of us are aware at the present time. We certainly recognize overt cases and do something about those. But sometimes it's very subtle. It is a matter of probing and knowing the right questions to ask and what to look for."

At HHAR, he also participates in the care of patients seen in some of their 130 monthly specialty clinics. "I am learning some of the particular entities that are seen in these clinics, whether ophthalmology (ear, nose, and throat) or dermatology." As well, he takes call at night with the on-call doctor to help manage the nursing home patients' emergencies as they arise. "At times, I am able to obviate the need for the transfer of a patient to an emergency department by providing care at HHAR. This eliminates the inherent 'transfer trauma' (both physical and psychological) that can accompany such a move."

Rounding out Michael's fellowship training is an eight-week intensive research methodology course, actually the very first rotation, followed by an ambitious research program in collaboration with Dr. Flomenbaum, who started the fellowship, and Dr. Sunday Clark, the emergency medicine research director at New York Presbyterian Hospital. Once he completes his fellowship year, Michael plans to remain at New York Presbyterian Hospital as an attending in the ED, and he will help direct the fellowship next year. "We have many very interested qualified applicants," he reports. Because this is a new fellowship, it is not yet accredited by ACGME [Accreditation Council for Graduate Medical Education]. "All fellowships start out this way," he explains. "It's our hope and belief that, especially given the response we have received so far, ultimately it will be accredited as a specific subspecialty of emergency medicine."

Michael's first career was as a professional artist, and his work was represented by a gallery in New York City. After 11 years as an abstract painter, he decided to pursue a career in medicine. He is beginning to paint again with water colors. "My history as an artist has helped me," he believes. "The ability to view a 'clinical picture' and see its elements has helped me as a diagnostician. There is a certain visual analysis that carries over into medicine and some of the hand–eye coordination that I learned while painting I can utilize while doing procedures." Agreeing that medicine is both a science and an art, Michael reports another person's observation that combining his work in emergency medicine and geriatrics is akin to being an archaeologist. He concurs, saying, "That would be a helpful description of what I'm doing: digging through the complex layers of geriatric medicine and picking out the jewels or gems that help us to learn how to better care for the elderly in the emergency setting. The only difference here is that there is still an opportunity to intervene and positively change the course of a patient's history while it is still important and before it is too late."

In his lecture presentations, Michael frequently intersperses major sections of his talk with some of the most famous paintings by leading artists throughout art history, including Michelangelo, Titian, Monet, Picasso, Matisse, Chagall, and O'Keefe. The works of art he highlights have all been created by the artists when they were over the age of 80 years old.

ENHANCING ELDER LIFE
IN HOSPITALS

Sharon K. Inouye, MD, MPH

As a young geriatrician caring for older patients at the bedside, Sharon K. Inouye, MD, MPH, recalls being struck by the poor outcomes of older patients. "Time and again I saw older people (usually age 70-plus) admitted to the hospital for acute problems and then, almost invariably, these people would do very poorly. Many developed cognitive and functional decline and ended up entering a nursing home. I asked myself, 'What is it that we are doing that causes hospital care to become almost toxic for an older person?' I wanted to explore the medications and procedures that might be contributing to the problem of delirium."

As a result of her experience, Dr. Inouye developed the Hospital Elder Life Program (HELP) during 1993–1994 at Yale University School of Medicine and tested it at Yale-New Haven Hospital (Inouye et al. 1999a, Inouye et al. 2000). The program was found to provide beneficial outcomes and to be cost-effective (Rizzo et al. 2001). Today, the model has been implemented in over 50 healthcare organizations nationally.

According to Dr. Inouye, delirium is an under-recognized but surprisingly common problem, particularly among older hospitalized adults. People who are delirious have trouble thinking clearly, focusing their thoughts, and paying attention. Delirium can appear suddenly over hours to days and may come and go during the course of a day. It can occur because the stresses of the hospital environment (such as medications, procedures, immobilization, and sleep deprivation) can overwhelm the adaptive responses of a vulnerable older person. Becoming delirious can be frightening; however, there are many ways that the problem can be prevented or properly handled. If left untreated, delirium can have serious consequences for recovery. Delirium is different from the long-term confusion seen with dementia or Alzheimer's disease. For more information refer to www.hospitalelderlifeprogram.org.

Dr. Inouye soon concluded that the current practice of hospital care for older adults was, in fact, contributing to their decline; a different way of approaching and caring for them became imperative. Dr. Inouye suggests that the treatment of older patients often is based on assumptions or protocols used for younger adults, without clear guidance by evidence or clinical indicators. "Often medications given routinely for sleep lead to confusion and delirium. Anti-ulcer medications are given routinely without a clear medical indication, and pain medications tend to be mismanaged in older persons," she reports.

"Another harmful approach involves the immobilization of older people in the hospital," Dr. Inouye relates sadly, "with no assessment of their ability to walk. They aren't allowed to get out of bed, and after bed rest for two or three days it becomes very difficult for an older person to walk. Indwelling bladder catheters are routinely inserted for no particular reason, unfortunately without assessment, often for the convenience of the staff.

"The underlying rationale for keeping older patients in bed was motivated by a fear that they might fall, the assumption being that an older, sick person needs to remain in bed, with no regard to how this negatively impacts the individual. A lack of education and inappropriate use of medication, along with overuse of bladder catheters, has led to immobilization. Unfortunately, such procedures adversely impact the well-being of an older person," explains Dr. Inouye.

Apart from harmful medical and clinical procedures, Dr. Inouye sees a fundamental negative attitude toward aging in our society that is also exhibited by healthcare providers. "Studies have documented that even though older patients may have many more medical problems than younger persons, the amount of time spent at the bedside by their healthcare providers is much less. Unfortunately, if the older patient is confused, the time spent decreases even more. Translating attitudes into time, a person's actions speak about the values we place on older people. We speak with our feet" (Inouye, Schlesinger, & Lydon 1999b).

As a Japanese–American, Dr. Inouye grew up in a cross-cultural and multigenerational family. "I always had an affinity for older persons," she relates. "Elders in the Japanese community find themselves honored as wise and cherished. When I became a healthcare provider, I witnessed how older people were being treated with an ageist approach. The novel *House of God* refers to old people as GOMERS ('get out of my emergency room'), a phrase that was quite popular when I was in medical school. During my training, I experienced such pervasive attitudes. I realized that elders represented an underserved segment of our population, with special, complex needs not being well addressed."

The HELP Program is not centered around a geriatric unit because such units serve only a small proportion of patients, according to Dr. Inouye. Instead, it serves patients hospital-wide, which is vital because 50% of all hospital beds are filled with people age 65 and older. In addition, the program does not use specialized geriatric teams moving from unit to unit diagnosing patients and making recommendations. "The problem with the geriatric consultation model," says Dr. Inouye, "is that the interventions recommended are often not carried out because the people on the receiving end of the counsel are not trained in geriatrics. For example, an orientation protocol (such as providing orientation boards and orienting communication) may be recommended for a patient, but the staff may be ill-equipped to conduct it. With HELP, the team makes and carries out the recommendations."

According to Dr. Inouye, HELP provides an organized system to actually do what everyone knows "should be done" in the care of older persons. The Geriatric Interdisciplinary Care team includes nursing, medicine, rehabilitation therapies, pharmacy, nutrition, and chaplaincy care as well as trained volunteers to provide support for patients and their families. The team also provides geriatric education programs for professional staff.

Dr. Inouye informs us, "The HELP program is also unique in the sense that it addresses six risk factors for delirium in older people:

- Daily volunteer visitation to provide orientation, cognitive stimulation, and social support for prevention of cognitive impairment;
- Early mobilization to prevent immobility;
- Use of a non-pharmacological sleep protocol, including massage and relaxation music, to prevent sleep deprivation;
- Hearing adaptations and equipment for the hearing impaired;
- Vision adaptations and equipment for vision impairment; and
- Encouragement of fluids to prevent dehydration."

Trained volunteers are an important part of the program because they help to bring a very human dimension to patients, notes Dr. Inouye. They conduct the orientation, mobility, and sleep protocol and assist with feeding and hydration. They also are involved in reminiscence activities, walking with patients, and other fun activities that keep patients mentally alert.

Extensively tested, HELP intervention resulted in:

- A significant reduction in the development of delirium and functional decline;
- Reduction in use and costs of hospital services, and the costs of implementing the program were offset by the cost savings realized from the program (Inouye et al. 1999; Inouye et al. 2000);
- A dose-response relationship between adherence to the interventions and delirium (Inouye et al. 2000);
- A reduction in use of long-term nursing home services and a 15.7% decrease in long-term nursing home costs, with an average savings of $9,446 per long-term nursing home patient (Leslie et al. 2005); and
- More people returned to their homes after hospitalization. Unfortunately, for economic reasons, the trend is to minimize hospitalization and transfer people from the hospital to a nursing home for rehabilitation. However, long-term residency has decreased because of HELP.

Dr. Inouye believes that the program positively impacts care provider attitudes. "In particular, the nursing staff views it as a way to help them deal with frail, confused, and difficult older patients," she underscores. "They represent our biggest supporters. It helps them to feel very good about the care they offer. And it helps to alleviate the pressures of being overworked."

Dr. Inouye reports that many of the hospital facilities embracing HELP expand the program to other populations including surgical, emergency room, and intensive care patients. She sees it eventually spreading to nursing homes and adult day care programs where HELP principles tend to be applicable.

"I believe our healthcare system must learn to deal with older people, because that is what the future brings," says Dr. Inouye, reflecting on the overall future of eldercare. "If we don't become good at caring for older people on principle, it will occur by necessity. I've been frustrated by the progress we've made in expanding HELP to a larger audience. The problems of delirium and functional decline of elders in hospitals are largely preventable and should be considered as quality indicators for hospital care. Systemically, older people are simply not being well cared for."

Continuing, she asserts, "People do not understand that geriatrics is just as different from average adult medicine as is pediatrics. You would never hear the latter being questioned, yet the differences between average adult medicine and geriatrics are equally great. Unfortunately, the number of geriatricians is quite small, and internists and other specialties do most of the care."

Dr. Inouye's sense of calling grew out of her family heritage, which included several generations of physicians, although only men. She recalls that while her grandmother was washing her hair one day when she was about six years old, her grandmother commented on the waste of having such a fine brain on a girl. "I knelt there in silence saying to myself that it was not a waste. I dedicated myself to go against the norm and to become a doctor and, literally hanging onto his leg, as a young child, demanded that my father include me every weekend in his rounds at the hospital."

Dr. Inouye's tenacity to follow her passion in the midst of such obstacles has led to her busy professional life. At the time of writing, Dr. Inouye served as the Director of the National HELP Dissemination Program, was a Professor of Medicine, Co-Director of the Yale Program on Aging and Claude D. Pepper Older Americans Independence Center, Director of the Yale Mentored Clinical Research Scholar Program, and Director of the Yale Mentorship Program in Patient-Oriented Research on Aging. She recently accepted new challenges as Professor of Medicine at Harvard Medical School, Milton and Shirley F. Levy Family Chair and Director of the Aging Brain Center at Hebrew Senior Life.

MERCY HEALTH CENTER

Christine H. Weigel, RN, BSN, MBA

One of the major benefits in becoming a Magnet™ facility is taking the journey to get there, believes Chief Nursing Officer Chris Weigel. "In striving for excellence, we looked at everything we were doing, with the objectives of determining how to be more efficient and have better outcomes for our patients."

Established by the American Nurses Credentialing Center (ANCC), a division of the American Nurses Association, Magnet is the highest award an organization can receive for nursing care. Held as the gold standard for nursing and patient care, Magnet status is awarded to those healthcare organizations demonstrating the best of nursing and patient care through adherence to international nursing professional standards.

Chris acknowledges the increasing number of elderly patients. "Caring for the elders needs to be part of our mission and services. We should care for elders with dignity and stewardship by taking time with patients and not rushing their care. Our objective should be service excellence. If that means a nurse taking a few minutes to sit with the patient, then we, as administrators, should be comfortable with that perspective."

Mercy Health Center in Oklahoma City is one of seven Sisters of Mercy Health System hospitals. Chris believes that the hospital has made great strides in addressing the needs of hospitalized elders. "We have especially addressed their needs relative to our physical environment. For example, we purchased new beds that have floor-level lights so patients can see when they get up at night. In addition, every acute care patient receives screening to determine whether they might be a candidate for a fall. If so, we put certain measures in place to minimize this possibility. Our new beds are in extra-low positions so that people can get in and out of them more easily. Also, if a person is at risk for falling, a magnet reading 'LAMP—Look At Me Please' is fixed to the door, reminding staff to peek in the room to make sure he/she is secure."

Chris informs us that they have moved to becoming a restraint-free facility. If patients appear confused at times and are likely to get up and hurt themselves, Mercy asks either a nursing assistant, volunteer, or family member to sit with them. Apparently, more and more healthcare environments are moving in this direction.

Chris states, "Hospitals are increasingly concerned about medication reconciliation. Elderly patients seem to be on more medications. We need to know all about the various medications, their interaction, and dosages, asking the attending doctor to reconcile any issues. We actually scan the medications at the bedside using the Bridge system. All medications have a bar code, and all patients have arm bands with an identifier to their list of medications. The nurse then scans the patient's name into the system before the medications are delivered. If the medications to be administered don't match existing data, the nurse is alerted. Since implementing the system, there have been no medication errors reported. Also, patients take home with them a written list of medications with instructions that are also reconciled."

To help staff develop a greater sensitivity in caring for the elderly, the hospital put together a learning packet of information created in-house. It addresses age-specific caring behaviors related to the elderly as well as to the very young and is reviewed annually. According to Chris, nurses in training often learn relative to the average age of a patient, but not necessarily things that are specific for the very young and very old. "With respect to the elderly, for example," she explains, "we want nurses to be aware of how to communicate with someone who is hard-of-hearing or who has dementia. They also need to understand that the tactile sensation of someone who is older is different and that we need to provide care a little slower."

The hospital also addresses the emotional and spiritual needs of patients. "We enjoy a very strong pastoral care program, with chaplains visiting every patient," Chris relates. "They serve as the eyes and hands for the nurses. We also have a strong social services component that helps with many of the emotional needs and changes relative to elderly patients having to leaving their homes and not being able to return immediately or not at all."

Mercy also participated in a study to learn how much time nurses or other caregivers spend at the bedside, almost a time-and-motion exploration. A number of hospitals were involved in the study, and Mercy was one of the first. The study looked at how much time nurses spent in documentation and in getting other resources and equipment necessary to carry out their duties. The objective involved determining how to increase the time spent at the bedside and how to design an environment that addresses the needs of both patient and caregiver. "I've seen some research indicating that nurses will walk close to five miles during a shift," Chris informs us. "We are fortunate to have a Nurse Server System with closets outside of each patient room containing the routine things needed every day."

Another concern is that as the population ages, the average age of a nurse increases as well. According to Health Resources and Services Administration (HRSA), in March 2004 the average age of the RN population was estimated to be 46.8 years of age, and according to the Government Accounting Office (GAO-01-944), 40% of all nurses will be older than age 50 by 2010 (www.gao.gov/cgi-bin/getrpt?GAO-01-944) (accessed July 30, 2006). Aware of these statistics, Chris reports that the hospital is committed to caring for their older nurses so that they don't experience burnout and they can be retained. "The entire system of buying equipment that is a help to them must be considered," she says. "For example, the new beds that we purchased both inflate and deflate on the sides, so that the nurse doesn't need to pull in order to turn a patient. In addition, it becomes vital to redesign units so the nurse doesn't need to walk as much. Our lifting equipment is appreciated as our population gets heavier. And, knowing that older nurses have difficulty in working 12-hour shifts, we work with flexible schedules.

"Achieving Magnet status doesn't mean you are perfect," Chris cautions. "Many hospitals provide excellent service but don't wish to invest the time required to engage in the process. It takes time to document and tell your story. However, we believe one of the major benefits at Mercy relates to the pride that the nurses and other staff feel in being a Magnet organization. Striving to become a Magnet facility was a good decision for us, and I think has contributed to our low staff vacancy rate of only 3–4%."

Looking For the Gaps in Eldercare

Suyrea Reynolds, NHA

Suyrea's career in caring for the elderly has been filled with challenges. She is a nursing home administrator (NHA) in Orlando, Florida, and also serves on Florida's Board of Nursing Home Administrators. She was hired by a hospital system seven years ago to develop a long-term care diversion program. "The diversion program was a pilot project with the state which required a Medicare HMO [health maintenance organization] partner. However, just as we were ready to sign a contract with the state, the company decided to no longer be in the Medicare HMO business." Although the original project was eliminated, she since has held multiple jobs with the hospital system, all centered on the elderly.

"I am one of two people in the organization who knows about nursing home administration," she acknowledges. "My whole career has been spent identifying the gaps in the continuum of care, always looking for what can be done next. My philosophy is that each elder is someone's baby girl or baby boy. It doesn't matter if they are old and frail or young with HIV [human immunodeficiency virus]. Someone loved them, I hope, when they were babies. That's what keeps me looking for what else we can do. In fact, the executive director of the hospital maintains the same focus. Over time, we have continued to look for the gaps in the continuum of care. My current position, which has been in place for the last two years, addresses this issue and is the only one of its kind that I know of with the sole purpose of this goal."

Suyrea concentrates on encouraging collaboration among the various interdisciplinary units that serve elders. "It's important that there is good collaboration between the nursing home doctor, hospital doctor, and services that are outside the acute care system such as psychiatry or ventilator care." As Suyrea explains, improving the continuum of care by enhancing collaboration between caregivers doesn't necessarily mean increased costs.

"Two years ago," Suyrea relates, "we found that our top physicians could be better utilized if they had physician extenders working with them in various aspects of elder care. Although these extenders originally reported to me, today they are out on their own. This is a good example of the way I like to work. I like to start programs, then turn responsibility of the program to another team member, allowing me time to find the next gap in the continuum that requires attention.

"Another gap in care was addressed when we heard from orthopedic surgeons who said that when their patients left the nursing home, often they had no therapy or home care until they went back for a checkup after their discharge. That's not good, because if you don't keep a knee or hip moving, it's going to freeze. We already had a program in place where a physical therapist (PT) meets with a patient prior to orthopedic surgery, visits the home to do an environmental assessment, and recommends appropriate changes such as removing rugs or getting an appropriate chair. The PT explains what will happen during surgery and answers questions. Now, we have another PT who visits patients while they are in the hospital, answers questions after surgery, then continues to follow the patient as the patient moves through the post-acute levels of care until the patient no longer requires therapy. In the process, we have been able to determine which facilities and home care organizations provide the best services."

Part of Suyrea's responsibilities involve setting up systems for hard-to-place patients. She enjoys a reputation of letting people know when competent service is being provided and where problems exist that need to be addressed. "Skilled nursing facilities know that when a nursing home provides excellent care, it will receive more referrals."

Another identified issue was follow-up care of young men and women who have newly acquired spinal cord injuries. After receiving rehabilitation, they return to their homes but then often returned to the hospital within a few weeks. "There is no half-way house for people with spinal cord injuries in our community," Suyrea explains. "So we developed a system to address the special at-home needs of a spinal-cord-injured individual. The Spinal Cord Program Coordinator just happens to be a quadriplegic who earned a master's degree after his accident and whose expertise involves working with those who have similar conditions. His job reinforces previous patient education, with the goal of making sure that these patients don't require readmission to the hospital. So many of these people are very angry and depressed," she reports. "Often individuals with new injuries are so overwhelmed with their state that they forget to shift their weight frequently, and quite often ulcers result. On a professional level, the coordinator bonds with these people, often reading them the riot act and reinforcing what the patient has learned during rehabilitation.

"I go nuts when a bad decision is made," she exclaims. "My job is to use my current position to pilot programs to meet identified needs. We have resource nurses in our hospital system and, at any given time, we can contact a clinical expert in pain or diabetes or infection control. We have used this model to develop a geriatric resource nurse designation, created a library and a curriculum, and will soon offer a two-day seminar to prepare acute care nurses for the gerontological nurse certification exam by the American Nurses Credentialing Center. Our registered nurses earn points towards increased salary by serving as an expert resource for their peers. Our goal is to have a geriatric resource nurse on every unit and every shift. And the key remains," Suyrea emphasizes, "that we offer this level of expertise without adding any staff!"

Suyrea's work serves as just one example of how looking for the gaps in healthcare service and filling them can not only enhance care, but also can diminish hospital-related inpatient expenses. It also demonstrates the many ways that administrators care for patients without being involved in hands-on service. "My job is to put my own needs to one side while exploring what can be done to support the staff," Suyrea underscores. "If I can help meet their needs, then they can meet the needs of the patient."

CARRIER OF THE LIGHT
IN HOSPICE CARE

Donna Brook, RN

"The whole system of taking care of our elders has to be reconstructed," Donna Brook, RN, says firmly. "We have to develop some kind of resources for people to take care of family members in their own homes. So often when people age, they find themselves in an environment where they are removed from a lifetime of memories. The food they eat is often not to their liking, and we force them into activities that they may never have been interested in pursuing."

As a hospice nurse, Donna admits the frustration she feels at times with the system. "But," she says, "I stay in the profession because I see myself as the carrier of the light; someone has to carry the light. You can see the difference you make in someone's life."

This concept of "light" resides at the core of Donna's hospice work, connecting the many parts with the whole. To "enlighten" means to brighten, change, alter, and illuminate. "Two of the most important attributes of hospice nursing are advocacy and education," she believes. "I cannot think of another arena of nursing where we educate not only the patient, but families and the medical community at large. Advocacy is critical because someone must speak out for the people who can't speak for themselves. When we speak out in this manner, we tend to lighten people's burdens."

"The hospice movement is relatively new in the United States," explains Donna, "and many people don't know what hospice involves. Or, they may have a misconception that it is appropriate during the last few days of life. Ideally, hospice should be provided during the last six months of life." Donna works for Comprehensive Community Hospice, a department in a skilled nursing facility in Lake Success, New York. Because of the setting, more than 90% of their hospice population tends to be elderly, defined as over 65, she notes. "In the nursing facility, roughly 60% of the people we serve are experiencing the end stages of dementia, Parkinson's Disease, or some other non-specific diagnosis. Because our technology is so advanced, we have many different ways of keeping people alive, so many people with dementia are living into their eighties and nineties. Unfortunately, there isn't the kind of hope that exists with cancer patients who may decide to engage in different treatment plans. The dementia patients we see basically fall into two categories, the first being those who come for a very short period of time, perhaps only for a week because the doctor doesn't think to make a referral earlier or the family members are ambivalent about making the move. On the other hand," she states, "we have dementia patients coming to us who continue living for a year or more. We view these patients as having a mysterious kind of resolve, attempting to survive even given their physical status. As long as they continue to meet the hospice criteria, we persist in serving them."

Relating to a dementia patient in a meaningful way as compared to someone whose mental abilities are normal can happen, believes Donna. "A nurse recently asked me, 'What are you really doing for these people? It's not like a cancer patient with whom you can communicate.' But we are communicating with them! Even though they may not communicate with words, I truly believe that at some level these patients understand that someone cares for them. We've noticed something very interesting. We find that some patients stabilize and improve after a period of time. Because they then no longer meet the hospice criteria, we face the dilemma of having to discharge them. I really believe that the attention and caring that the patients receive ameliorates the course of their disease. Regrettably, after discharge, they often regress and fail to thrive. It's a paradox universal to hospice programs. We often feel that we are abandoning them."

According to Donna, the typical indicator for admission to hospice is the failure to thrive resulting from repeated infections or weight loss caused by clenching their teeth and not eating. But, when they enter hospice, they experience a different environment. "Our hospice providers are trained and motivated to engage with patients whatever their condition. Nurses, certified nursing aides, social workers, and spiritual care people pay attention to them. We work our magic and suddenly there is a will to live."

Donna has any number of stories to illustrate "working our magic." She tells the delightful story of a little 95-year-old old lady with dementia who had been living at home with a very caring family and who had hired some private help to care for her. At one point, she totally stopped eating and became extremely disengaged. "She eventually came to hospice and we served her for almost a year," Donna recounts. "One of her nurses was a male who usually delivered her sleeping medication. Within a period of a few months, she began to eat again to at one point getting herself out of bed, walking to the kitchen, and eating an entire cake. She improved to the degree of gaining weight and being able to engage more with the staff and with her family. Her whole status changed which, of course, was quite confusing to the family."

Coping with such frustrations can be difficult for staff to process. Consequently, a facilitator conducts monthly support sessions for the Community Hospice staff. In addition, as a relatively small, cohesive group, the staff functions like a family, engaging in social activities outside the office as well.

"Hospice involves an enormous amount of education," Donna explains. "When we first established our program seven years ago, we had one or two referrals from our parent facility, whereas today we might have at least 20 patients. Yet still, even more people should be referred to us. So, we plug along and know that we are making a difference. We see it in our patients and also hear it from their families, that without our services a person's remaining time on earth might be much different."

Donna sees some people at the end of their lives who are consumed with regret for all of the things they wanted to do but didn't. They may express anger, guilt, or resentment and haven't dealt with the issues surrounding such feelings. These feelings tend to come to the surface when a person is dying. "That's really sad," she reflects caringly. "I remember going to a conference on the dying process and hearing the poet John O' Donahue mentioning that the greatest regret is a life unlived.

"People nearing the end of their life often engage in a life review process, remembering all of the things they've said and done in their lives. Unfortunately, some people become very frightened. I've had patients who have regretted a particular action and are fearful, perhaps because of a particular belief system about heaven and hell. For this reason, it is vital that people engage in a process of forgiveness, especially self-forgiveness, which is not necessarily religious in nature."

Donna also talks about the clients who are an inspiration to the staff. Donna fondly remembers a very interesting lady with colon cancer, which had spread throughout her body, who had died recently. "She was simply adorable," Donna recalls. "She was a tiny wisp of a person, she was about 98 years old, probably five feet tall, and weighed around 80 pounds. Emigrating from Ireland, she had been married for about forty years and then widowed for a similar period of time. When she entered hospice, they gave her about one week to live, but she remained in our program for almost a year. She loved to tell dirty jokes, regardless of who came to visit her. Sometimes we as service providers visiting her might think that we were having a bad day. But by the time we left we found ourselves laughing, because she had the most incredible sense of humor. She would just light up, hold your hand, and thank you for taking care of her, even though she was experiencing pain because of the cancer. It was like being in the presence of an astonishing person."

Sharing an example of how she uses her visionary skills during her work with hospice patients, she tells the story of John (not his real name). "I have a really wonderful example, although this man was younger," she states. "John had been involved in our program for about nine months. Two of us often visited him because he mumbled his words. One of us would read his lips while the other took notes. At one point, he mentioned having been an avid sailor. He loved the beach and really wished he could be there again. After leaving his house one day, the two of us spontaneously visited a boating store. We said to ourselves, 'Why not take a sailboat and the beach to John?' At the store, right on the top of the counter, we spotted a painting of a beach, complete with sand and umbrella. We really got carried away and the next time we visited John we came loaded with sand, a candle with a summer aroma, water, and music. A look of peace came over John and for the first time he agreed to a Reiki session. The following week, his spirit was lifted so much that he decided he didn't need hospice any more." Here we have another example of Donna and her colleagues utilizing "vision" and working their magic.

We suspect that one of the biggest challenges related to hospice care involves working with patients who enter with a sense of hopelessness, giving up any expectation of surviving and thriving. However, Donna informs us that what people don't understand about hospice is that it is not a place but a philosophy. You don't come two days before you die. Hospice workers care with great dedication, but not with the expectation that they are going to cure a person. "We expect to maximize their quality of life for whatever period of time that is left," she exclaims. "What I find really interesting with patients is that sometimes those who say that they don't want to go through the chemo and radiation may live longer and have more quality of life than those who continue with treatments until the end. So it often doesn't involve giving up, but trusting that there will be quality of life and even a good death."

Comprehensive Community Hospice uses several nonclinical therapy modalities, including Reiki, Therapeutic Touch, and aromatherapy. In addition, one of the doctors is an Ayurvedic practitioner, an Indian-based system using many different herbal remedies. According to Donna, these tend to be much safer than some of the Chinese herbs, and he uses them holistically to treat problems such as appetite and nausea in the cancer population.

For the families of hospice patients, Donna recommends a book entitled *Gone From My Sight—A Dying Experience*, giving them a sense of what it means to be involved in the process of dying (Karnes 2001). People find it enormously helpful. It's a very soothing little book supporting the concept that death is a transition (see the poem at the end of this section).

The current models of caring for elders must be changed, Donna believes, re-emphasizing her initial comments on reconstructing eldercare. "The money that we spend in nursing homes is sinful. Eldercare is so much more than handing out pills and filling up feeding tubes. Many nursing homes seem to be terribly disengaged from genuine caring. We are not allowing people to continue living their lives. Nursing homes tend to be so regimented that they operate more like jails then homes. People often find themselves sitting in wheelchairs in the hallways watching talk shows on television, just sitting and waiting to die. And yet," she says, "there is some hope, because there are facilities that are changing the way they look and their approach to elders and their care."

We heartily concur with Donna's perception, which serves in part as the motivating force behind this book. In addition, we believe that the reconstruction of eldercare must begin, as Donna suggests, with a reoriented belief system and philosophy about aging, perhaps best summarized by the words of Eleanor Roosevelt: "Beautiful people are accidents of nature, but beautiful old people are works of art."

I am standing upon the seashore.
A ship at my side spreads her white sails to the morning breeze and starts for the blue ocean.

She is an object of beauty and strength.
I stand and watch her until at length she hangs like a speck of white cloud just where the sea and sky come to mingle with each other.

Then someone at my side says: "There, she is gone!"

"Gone where?"

Gone from my sight. That is all.
She is just as large in mast and hull and spar as she was when she left my side and she is just as able to bear her load of living freight to her destined port.

Her diminished size is in me, not in her.
And just at the moment when someone at my side says:

"There, she is gone!" there are other eyes watching her coming, and other voices ready to take up the glad shout:

"Here she comes!"

And that is dying.

—Henry Van Dyke

Bridging Troubled Waters

Nancy Merrill, Improving Care Program Assistant

M any people are familiar with end-of-life programs such as hospice. Often, however, people who may be declining in health find themselves in between services—not yet diagnosed as being terminal and eligible for hospice, but not fully functioning as they did formerly. A few programs attempt to meet their needs.

Improving Care Through the End of Life, sponsored by Franciscan Services in Tacoma, Washington, is one such program. Designed as a bridge between a diagnosis and hospice care, its goal is to help patients nearing the end of their lives make informed choices with dignity, understand all of their medical options, and be aware of what they can expect as their illness progresses. Because Improving Care programs are based in community medical clinics, they can typically connect with patients whose illness was recently diagnosed but who have not yet reached a point of crisis. By getting to know patients at this early juncture, there is time to help them make thoughtful, informed choices that reflect their wishes and values.

According to Nancy Merrill, Improving Care Program Assistant at Enumclaw Medical Clinic, Enumclaw, Washington, the program's objective is to connect families with community services, enabling their family member to remain at home and creating better communication between patients and physicians. "In essence, we serve as the patient's advocate and liaison with community services and healthcare resources," she explains. "A nurse makes an initial assessment and gains an understanding from the patient about his/her condition and their caregiving issues. We also ask the individual's physician a series of questions to help the physician determine the patient's appropriateness for Improving Care. One of the questions asked is, 'Would you be surprised if this patient died in a year?' If the answer is 'no,' then the patient is likely at risk for getting worse and may be referred to the Improving Care program."

Nancy says that patients on the program benefit from having a direct phone link to the nurse. Having a healthy level of trust established with the nurse makes asking questions easier. A chaplain is also available as needed. Eventually, when appropriate, the nurse can recommend hospice to the patient's physician and then to the patient.

"This alleviates some of the shock of being told that death will come sooner than later. Our program becomes an in-between safety net," she states.

Improving Care relies on trained volunteers who maintain regular contact with those in the program. "Volunteers call or visit people monthly and are trained to pick up on the red flags. Perhaps someone is having increasing difficulty with long-term pain or problems with balance," Nancy explains. "Many of these people find themselves dealing with a number of dependency issues, such as no longer being able to drive a car or perhaps cook a meal. Volunteers can help people deal with these losses through listening and alerting the nurse about emerging needs to be addressed. They may run errands for a patient, but most often, they serve as a friend."

Nancy's interest in end-of-life issues as a whole led her to her involvement with Honor My Wishes™, a community volunteer effort designed to enhance end-of-life conversations and help people understand the importance of making their own choices known. She serves as the president of the volunteer board. "Many people feel uncomfortable talking about end-of-life wishes with their families and loved ones. Honor My Wishes™ volunteers utilize the Respecting Choices© Advance Care Planning model of community outreach to train facilitators in churches and other community groups to help people initiate such conversations. The group recently developed an Honor My Wishes Personal End-of-Life Binder that helps individuals organize their wishes with regard to medical care, financial affairs, and final commemorating plans. The extensive binder provides information, sample forms, and ideas for imparting personal messages people may want to communicate to their families. The binder format allows for accumulating new information and can be used to keep important documents in one place. The goal of the group is for everyone in their community to have a binder. A grant from the Robert Wood Johnson Foundation Rallying Points covered the binder's design and the cost of an initial printing of 500. Thereafter, it is anticipated that people will obtain a binder for a nominal fee (www.honormywishes.org).

Weaving a Tapestry of Healthcare Resources

Cathleen Ingle, MSW

Bloomington Indiana Hospital and Healthcare System's Transitions Program began about six years ago, according to Cathleen Ingle, the program's coordinator. Transitions is a national model embracing more than 73 organizations in the United States. Bloomington adopted the program based on the hospice team's experience that a number of people came into hospice very near the end their lives, recalls Cathleen. Helping people to become comfortable at such a late stage and to get their needs met was rather challenging. "Apart from pain management, there is not a whole lot of physical intervention," she says, "but from emotional and spiritual perspectives, much can be accomplished."

The Transitions Program is designed to help people bridge the gap between being sick enough to be in the hospital, progressing through major treatment, until they become hospice appropriate. The challenge is how to help these people get to where they need to be to receive holistic care.

"Finding appropriate services can be challenging for a family," Cathleen states. "I counsel people to ask questions, especially of social workers. Probably no other healthcare professional exists who is a jack-of-all-trades, master of none, in terms of information and resources," she relates firmly. "Because we don't work with age or income guidelines in the Transitions Program, we find ourselves privileged to involve ourselves with entire family systems. Initially people often tell us that they don't need a social worker. But, when we get them to talk about their situation and what they do need, the conversation frequently extends to an hour or more. Our job is to fill in the gaps. Sometimes we think of ourselves as quilt makers, piecing together all of the scraps of the various resources and agencies. It's kind of an art. Because every person's needs are different, we attempt to create one whole tapestry by piecing together a variety of resources, beginning by helping them articulate a primary concern and then build from there. I can spend hours on the telephone negotiating services for people. Family members who are taking care of an elder simply do not have the time, knowledge, or stamina to do this kind of research."

Such a program serves as an excellent response to what gerontologists call "environmental press," the demands that social and physical environments make on people to adapt or change. In terms of elders, physical limitations emerge with age, and social support systems may become less available. The Transitions Program serves as one excellent example of how such environmental pressures can be relieved.

People enter the Transitions Program via referrals from healthcare providers, social workers, nurses, doctors, home healthcare workers, and community and family members. "Home care agencies are typically the most responsive and quick to refer," Cathleen notes. At the hospital, the highest number of people who can be served is about 40, and there is an extensive waiting list. Cathleen explains, "We must attempt to work with families, triaging people to determine who can be served best and most quickly. In addition, when a referral comes to us from someone other than from a physician, we contact the patient's doctor and explain our services. Often the physician is surprised about what we offer but pleased and glad to hear from us."

Even though the program is limited in scope, Cathleen works to see that every referral receives help in some form. "As a social worker, some ethical obligations must be embraced," she asserts. "We talk among ourselves in terms of doing what is right for a person. At a minimum, we provide information and referral services for people we are not going to be able to admit. Either over the phone, or during an initial home visit, we conduct an assessment and help people identify all of the resources of which they can avail themselves, although often these may be limited. At least a person will know about every waiting list offered by agencies on aging, their capacity, or whether the individual might be eligible for Medicaid and how to apply. They might be able to get prior authorization for some assistance at home."

The Transitions Program designs centers around helping people who are homebound, seeking to assist people in maintaining their quality of life and as much independence as is possible. It also serves as a bridge, assisting people to transition to the next level of care.

We speculate that as the population ages, more and more services will be required. Even prior to any type of intervention and treatment, people begin to develop problems such as diminishing mobility, loss of short-term memory, and perhaps emotional issues. Asked about the kinds of advice she might offer to families who have aging relatives, Cathleen responds, "It's not easy to answer that question. First, it is important to educate oneself about Medicaid and know how it differs from Medicare. Medicare does not have to be as intimidating as it sounds. I always tell people to pay attention to the breadth of home health coverage, looking for changes and little nuances in the language regarding reassessment and medication. The task is to keep asking; there are no silly questions."

Second, Cathleen underscores the importance of people being gentle with themselves and not getting caught up in the "shoulds and oughts" of caregiving. "In reality, caregiving is often challenging, gut-wrenching, and physically exhausting. On the other hand, it can be fun and enjoyable, creating precious moments."

Cathleen also emphasizes the importance of respite self-care, which is why volunteers play an important role in the Transitions Program. "Two hours doesn't sound like much time," she asserts, "but it allows people to get some sleep, take a shower, or simply sit under a tree in the back yard and do nothing. No matter how much we give care and nurturance to another, there isn't a single person who doesn't need personal time off before reengaging. Many people perceive this as a luxury, but it must be seen as a fundamental, personal need. It sounds so simple, but often it is a hard truth to grasp, and to disengage as a caregiver without feeling guilt can be extremely difficult. We call it guilt-free rest."

Cathleen fills two roles—her professional job and as part of the family caring for her elderly grandmother. Taking care of herself becomes doubly important. "I'm extremely fortunate to have this job; it's the best one ever, especially because of the working environment," she says. "I'm not talking about office space, which is cramped and insufficient," she reminds us, "but there is always support; there is someone with whom you can discuss a case or process an issue. We have an interdisciplinary team that listens to each other and works together. We enjoy an excellent holistic clinical atmosphere, which is vital because we are affected by every client with whom we work, so we are allowed to laugh, cry, and sometimes scream."

The staff has a number of nonclinical resources available, including having a bereavement luncheon periodically. "Once every three months, we gather in a community room of a local mortuary where we talk personally about our patients we cared for and the impact they have had upon our lives. We discuss what we need to do to take care of ourselves so we can continue to support others. The chaplain offers spiritual support. And we always read the names of the people we have cared for and often include the joy we have received from them. It becomes a very healing event."

Along these lines, we highly recommend a delightful, little book by Elaine Childs-Gowell, ARNP, PhD, entitled *Good Grief Rituals*. It is filled with imaginative, yet practical, tools and healing rituals for letting go of grief (Childs-Gowell 1992).

There is also an employee health fitness center, and people have the opportunity of talking with the psychiatrist on staff. "We can talk with her at any time about the challenges of our job; it's a safe place to do that. Whether or not we utilize that resource, sometimes it's helpful just knowing that it is available," Cathleen affirms.

Another important self-care practice involves the ability to utilize humor. Cathleen believes that you can't be an effective healthcare provider without laughter as well as tears, both of which are vital components of emotion and passion. "Sometimes we tell ourselves that we are crazy because we work here," she laughs. "When people become superstressed, some people get snappy; some of them cry; but when I'm totally overloaded and at my limit, I feel uncontrollable laughter erupting up in me, often accompanied with tears streaming down my face! It only happens once in a great while and the only thing to do is to roll with it. Otherwise, you can't function. It's part of the work environment."

Cathleen depends on the support of her good friends away from her work environment, and the enjoyment she finds in creative writing is one of her important outlets. She seldom goes home at the end of the day without processing its events. She reports, "I can't always fix a problem. But I absorb a lot, so when entering a home, sometimes I come out like a drippy sponge. It's not OK for me to go home with my stress mess and drip all over my family and pets. So, the place to do this is with colleagues. First, it is a matter of confidentiality and, secondly, they just get it. You don't have to work hard to explain the situation. If we don't meet in person, at least we talk on our cell phones."

Some people would describe this as connecting to community. We believe connecting to community stands foremost in the hierarchy of the self-care strategies.

To fill this need for community building in a more structured way in the healing professions, Rachel Naomi Remen, MD, created a program called Finding Meaning in Medicine, establishing support groups for healthcare workers. A free (you must register first) Resource Guide Starter Kit is available at www.meaninginmedicine.org. A free support group facilitator's guide is also available by contacting us at jlhenry@aol.com.

No matter how much energy she puts into her work, Cathleen believes that her clients and their families give back a thousandfold. "It is a privilege to associate with people who are nearing the end of their lives. They have a limited amount of time and physical/emotional resources, yet they connect with us," she says emotionally. "We find ourselves engaging in a small part of their journey. What a true gift we are given through these intimate occasions. My supervisor, Jan, likens it to birth. We get to be with them on their way out."

Cathleen often experiences the reality that many elders simply say what they think without making apologies or worrying about other people's reactions. It's "What you see is what you get." They portray a level of humanity rarely found elsewhere. "I have a gentleman with Alzheimer's whom I simply adore," she shares feelingly. "I didn't know him before he fell into dementia. He is funny and a little bit of a flirt; he always grabs my hand and tells me he loves me. He simply exudes joyfulness. His wife affirms that he had always been this way, but now he experiences living without worries. It comes back to honesty—honesty from older people that you don't find elsewhere.

"The other vital reality, whether using the word or not, involves having a healthy sense of spirituality. Whatever one's perception might be of a higher power, we must be tuned into it. Just yesterday I helped a 42-year-old woman tell her 16-year-old daughter that she was dying with cancer. She did it beautifully, but her daughter still didn't quite get it. I said to myself, 'Please God, help this child, because I can't do anything more for this family. It is in your hands.' I am a conduit through which energy flows."

Cathleen's comments remind us that the word "health" is derived from the old Saxon word "hal," meaning "whole." Just so, when we say "hello" to another person we mean we hope they are hal or whole. Just as the human body functions as an organic whole, we cannot afford to exclude the psycho/social/spiritual dimensions of our being.

Asked to describe a more perfect, holistic eldercare system, Cathleen says, "Physically, I don't know what it would look like. However, it would be some kind of a place that is not agency-centered, perhaps more like a life cycle continuum that is not sterile and not difficult to access. It would be more like a clearinghouse of information where people could connect with each other, where people who have been caregivers could impart their wisdom to those just beginning their work. Often, caregivers remain isolated from one another, and there is nothing more debilitating than to be inaccessible to others."

In today's typical medical model, care for elders often is often less than optimal. While Cathleen has tremendous respect for the work of physicians, she believes that unfortunately they often view a patient's reality from the perspective of a 15- or 20-minute office visit, a viewpoint that can be less than holistic. "I believe that we need to do a better job of educating our physicians about caring for elders and their special issues," she says emphatically.

For example, Cathleen explains that compared to the overall population, percentage wise, more elders experience depression than other segments of the population, and doctors may be prone to treat it with medications. Often, however, depression can be linked to grieving over a loss, loneliness, isolation, or anxiety, and therefore may be treatable in other ways. Consequently, physicians need improved education regarding the vital role all other healthcare providers play.

A more holistic approach to health care would include an understanding and treatment of emotional, psychological, and spiritual as well as physical discomfort. According to Cathleen, ideally, elders would have access to an interdisciplinary team of healthcare providers including a family practice physician, geriatric specialist, oncologist, social worker, chaplain, nurse, home health aide, geriatric psychiatrist, pharmacist, physical therapist, occupational therapist, and massage therapist.

Being a caring person begins with honesty, Cathleen believes. "Caring is not about putting a Band-Aid on a situation or simply handing out resource pamphlets," she says. "Or, if there are no resources available for the person, caring involves telling the truth and seeking to identify alternatives. True caring is genuine," she states firmly. "The motivation behind it has nothing to do with increasing one's patient satisfaction score or with bringing more referrals to your agency."

REMEMBERING PAPAW

Francie Horn, LCSW, CCBT, BCD

"Papaw was probably in his eighties when I met him in the hollows of West Virginia," recalls Francie Horn fondly. "The family's story represents one of the greatest experiences and joys I've had in my work with elders. An Alzheimer's patient, Papaw had 15 adult children whose ages spanned 32 years. With that much age difference, I naturally assumed that there were two moms; but no, I was told there was only one mother who had been killed four years earlier when she was run over by a tractor-trailer. What struck me," says Francie, "was the enormous sense of community and support that his adult kids had for their father. It was phenomenal. They took turns taking care of him. He did not want to go into a nursing home, nor did they want him to. He would wander at times and was confused, though he was never aggressive. He was interested in his family, making it clear that he was still their father; he knew best and they shouldn't forget it.

"You can only imagine the challenges of working with this family. Three daughters had the same name, so I had to be very politically correct in how I asked which one was calling me," Francie laughs. "There was a lot of humor involved from both ends, with family members being able to laugh at themselves as well as chiding me for not understanding life in the hollow. It was all done in good humor and fun. The respect they had for their father was amazing. Whenever we had a care conference, everyone came. I did multiple interventions, whatever was needed at the time, including helping a couple of the younger ones with substance abuse and getting services for one of Papaw's children who was severely autistic. I provided a lot of education about Alzheimer's disease, and I interacted with community agencies to get him services and some adaptive equipment so that he could remain in the home. I became the entire family's advocate over the two years I worked with them."

Francie currently works as a Board Certified Licensed Clinical Social Worker/ Psychotherapist at Orlando Regional Healthcare in Orlando, Florida. Francie's caseload and her private practice include both elderly and non-elderly disabled adults. She appreciates the interdisciplinary team of nurses, physicians, case managers, and aides with whom she works, helping patients deal with the acute healthcare challenges they are facing.

Many of the patients Francie sees are in their sixties to nineties in four inpatient cardiac units; they may have had by-pass surgery, a valve replacement, or a heart attack. "It's a very emotional time for people who have had a heart attack or who are facing major surgery. Their coping mechanisms may be stretched thin; they may be grieving over losing their sense of independence. I also see patients in a monitored unit where people may have experienced acute chest pain and are then admitted to rule out myocardial infarction (heart attack) and to determine the etiology of their chest pain. I see everything from people with substance and alcohol abuse to the elderly living alone without a support system. Then, of course, there are always the family dynamics to deal with. People have different coping mechanisms," she explains. "They may be depressed and anxious. Their control has been taken away. Elderly people often have accumulated losses over the course of many years, and their own physical problems may trigger the feelings associated with those losses, such as the death of family members, even the loss of a job or retirement that hasn't worked out, all of which impact medical outcomes and recovery," she relates. Consequently, she spends considerable time educating the nurses on the units about the impact that depression, anxiety, grief, loss, and being alone, isolated without a support system, have on a patient's health and recovery.

In working with patients, Francie can get a sense of whether spirituality is the patient or the family's focus of strength. "I usually ask about their spirituality or religious beliefs, although I never talk religion," she notes. "I can usually get people to talk about their spirituality when they are in a medical crisis. I just bring it to the forefront. Spirituality has a great impact on the patient's coping mechanisms and subsequent recovery." Spirituality is different from religion, she believes. Some people believe in God or angels, and many believe they have guardian spirits, says Francie. "Sometimes my patients will ask me to pray with them; I always ask whether they would like a visit from a chaplain. At times, the chaplain's and my role intertwine," she explains.

As a country, the kind of support and services offered to the elderly varies significantly from state to state, according to Francie. Some states do a good job, while others offer very few services, many of which are only on paper because funding doesn't keep pace with the needs of elders. In some cases, people needing services may have to wait up to three years. "I've worked in five states as a social worker and can attest to how varied the in-home to community-based services and benefits are."

Given such variation, Francie agrees that people contemplating moving to another state after retirement should find out what benefits the state offers and whether there is a lengthy waiting list for services. "I do think that baby boomers won't put up with the difficulties their parents may have faced in accessing home and community services. They won't sit back and take someone's word, but will get on the Internet and educate themselves about their options. Although we've made big strides in helping our elders, we have a ways to go," she states emphatically.

Francie is an innovator, explaining, "I always use multiple and multimodal interventions, using/implementing unusual adaptive equipment—Windsor Feeder, the Diana Lift, HandiLift, for example—and try to get funding from state or other funding sources in order to help patients remain at home as long as possible. This is *always* in addition to getting them local and state entitlement programs and services such as in-home community-based services for housekeepers, home health aides, and transportation to doctor appointments or shopping.

"For example, I had an elderly woman who was alert and well-oriented, but who had functional deficits causing her to be in a wheelchair. She wanted to remain in her home for as long as possible; fortunately, she had the funds to hire a private caregiver, but for only four hours a day. I was able to get the Windsor Feeder for her, which her caregiver would set up for her every day ahead of the time for dinner, which allowed her to eat at her own pace and without assistance. I also got the HandiLift paid for by the State of Florida (only after many months of advocacy!). The state paid for installation so that tracks for the Lift went from her bed to bathroom and into the living room. This allowed her to get out of bed by herself, or with minimal assistance, and into her wheelchair on her own and also go to the bathroom and/or shower. It was a phenomenal task but well worth the 'fight' to get the adaptive equipment she needed. I wish I could say that this was the norm as far as success went, but I always feel that if I'm able to help one person, then it's always a success, in my mind."

Continuing, she remarks, "With demented patients who are psychotic, having hallucinations and delusional thinking, in order to decrease or prevent catastrophic reactions, I use a host of interventions from my 'bag of tricks.' If one approach won't work, I'll keep trying other modalities until something does work.

"Keep in mind that the following interventions were done in the late 1980s and early 1990s, *before* we knew much about the etiology of dementia and *before* interventions like these were acceptable. In fact, during those years, I was really going against the trend. It was common for staff in nursing facilities catering to demented people to do 'reality orientation,' which doesn't work for moderate to late-stage dementia. "I had a patient in the nursing home who was hallucinating, believing there were bugs in her room. No amount of attempting to convince her otherwise worked. So I instructed the staff to go into her room with plastic bottles of water and tell her that they were spraying the bugs with pesticide; they sprayed all around the baseboards in her room and, behold, her hallucinations stopped.

"Another demented patient living in her own home was obsessed that her ex-husband was stalking her with an intent to kill her. I got permission from the home health care director to have a male nurse from the agency come to visit her (I was present); he pretended that he was a policeman and said that her ex-husband had been arrested (luckily, they had been divorced for over 20 years and he lived in another state) and that he would never bother her again. Her delusions and hallucinations completely disappeared and never returned."

Francie is also certified in some modalities of energy medicine/psychology, e.g. Thought Field Therapy, that are useful with elderly patients who have difficulty expressing their emotions or who don't want conventional counseling. Energy medicine is useful for helping to decrease depressive, obsessive, and anxious symptoms as well as trauma and loss.

Services for the elderly today are too fragmented, and families don't know where to go for help nor what questions to ask, believes Francie. "I would create a one-stop shopping organization, if you will, where a person's cognitive, physical, and support system needs would be assessed from an interdisciplinary perspective. Keeping people in their homes is cheaper, even when they need some assistance or adaptive equipment and family member training, than the cost of being in a nursing home, which can cost upwards of $5,000 a month, which may not include the cost of their medications and therapies." Admittedly, dealing with limited available resources and services is frustrating. Yet, Francie chooses to remain in her profession. "I think what sustains me is the belief that if I am able to help even one person, that's enough. Rarely do you get thanked, so the work has to be its own gratification.

"Listening is the biggest gift you can give someone," affirms Francie. "Listening is empowering; it enables people and recognizes what their strengths and differences are. I hope that is the gift that we give the elders with whom we work. I learn so much from the elders I meet," she states. "I admire their strength and perseverance in addition to their high value system and ethics. For many, life was hard, not just medically. They have had hardships, and yet they have persevered. Their strength and high ethical standards in general are traits that I aspire to."

Acknowledging the importance of caring for self, Francie explains her own self-caring strategies. "Self-caring," she says, "includes continuing your own spiritual, personal growth, which gives us more insights into other people's experiences. Personally having broader experiences can help us to globalize other cultures and religions, transcending those barriers that may still exist." Francie also cares for herself through the use of her artistic skills. Multitalented, she plays the piano and composes songs, four of which have been copyrighted. She also enjoys arts and crafts and painting; she paints, mostly landscapes using acrylics, and won a third prize in the New Hampshire State Art Exhibition in 1990.

"GOING WITH THE FLOW"— CARING FOR THE ELDERLY

Jocelyn M. Porquez, NP, CS, APRN-BC

"Diminishing the true value of older adults in our western culture is a huge problem," believes Jocelyn Porquez, a board certified family nurse practitioner and psychiatric clinical nurse specialist. She has considerable experience as a consultant and in directing care for the aged in assisted living communities and nursing home facilities. Her area of clinical expertise centers on depression and dementia.

"One of my closest friends is an elderly priest who is about to retire and enter a retirement community. Recently, he said, 'I intend to end up in a facility designed for healthy people.'" In her practice, Jocelyn has observed that patients who have consistent family support tend to recover and improve from health crises at a faster rate than those without family support. These patients seem to feel encouraged to live each day more fully, inspired by the love for a child or grandchild, or in anticipation of a future special event. Active, with a sense of aliveness, they thrive. Without hope, their emotional and physical health seems to decline. A nursing home patient describes this phenomenon as living "in a quarantined dullness." In fact, one elderly man likens his experience in a nursing home to "living in a warehouse for old people waiting to die." In earlier years, he had been vibrant and successful in business, but now he has lost his desire to live.

Jocelyn is a Filipino–American, whose father is a successful general surgeon. They recently returned to the Philippines on a surgical–medical mission. "No assisted living or nursing homes exist in the Philippines," she explains. "There, elders are respected as a source of compassion, wisdom, and strength, and they care for them in their older years. It would be an embarrassment not to care for one's elders. It is considered a blessing to be able to give back to them what they nurtured and invested in us. Honored and respected elders living in third world countries are much happier and have more productive lives. In comparison, the American culture still prizes the corporate illusion of youth and vitality.

"My vision for healing is holistic, embracing an integrated biopsychosocial-spiritual model for health and well-being," Jocelyn says emphatically. She believes that our American culture is heavily influenced by the medical and pharmaceutical industry, which is directing us to reach for a different pill every time there is a newly encountered symptom.

"'Polypharmacy' can be dangerous to the elderly because their lowered metabolic rate slows the elimination and detoxification of potent medications," explains Jocelyn. "There can also be a variety of cross-drug interactions, which have serious side effects. Unfortunately, due to insurance policies and restrictions, many healthcare professionals are forced to just prescribe medications rather than pursue the best treatments available. It is not uncommon for the elderly to have multiple specialists and healthcare providers. This creates chaos and makes communication among the various healthcare professionals difficult. The elderly end up having no competent leadership who can effectively supervise their overall health care. Someone needs to address the elderly [person] as fully alive and whole, and not only as a specific organ system that needs a drug. Aliveness is about having energy. This is why I approach the body as essentially flowing energy. I have learned that illness occurs when there is a block in the natural flow of the body's energy. Energy blocks can be removed by helping people understand why they are trapped in reoccurring emotions and behavior patterns. By using new techniques to release these blocks, patients are given the opportunity for a new life and better relationships. It is humbling to see people's health and lives improve when I reveal to them the possibilities of living."

Unfortunately, "polypharmacy" is growing, according to Jocelyn. She strongly believes in the importance of good nutrition and in simplifying the medications that are prescribed by healthcare specialists. There are very few cases in which all the medications they are taking are necessary. "One of my roles," she explains "is to review all patients' medications along with their collaborating physicians and determine which medication may be eliminated. Many times patients may no longer require certain drugs. Elders need to be carefully monitored to determine if all of their medications are still necessary. My role serves as a 'pharmaceutical referee' for patients and their specialists. On an ongoing basis, I communicate and educate families about their loved one's progress. At times, I recommend discontinuing a patient's medications to determine their baseline requirements to see which ones are needed. In doing so, many times their health can improve over 20 to 30 percent. I also have found that delirium and depression can be the result of overmedication. It is possible to wean patients off certain medications and see them recapture their real selves again."

Jocelyn incorporates a number of new healing modalities in her work including stress management, meditation, good nutrition, and Neuro-Emotive Technique (NET). NET is a new method of finding and releasing energy blocks in the body called "neuro-emotional complexes" or NECs (see www.netmindbody.com). Often these NECs are caused by specific emotionally traumatic events in the past that are held onto by the body, causing blocks in the natural flow of its energy. NET identifies and removes these physiological and emotional blocks. A successful NET session causes a physiological change that can support long-lasting emotional health and transformation. Jocelyn is also using this approach with Jeff Pendergrast, MD, a plastic surgeon, who is transforming and rejuvenating patients both physically and emotionally. Together they are offering a new approach to physical and emotional well-being.

Aesthetic surgery is often an elective procedure for women who desire a dramatic change in their appearance and an improvement in their self-image. In rare instances, despite successful plastic surgery, a woman may not feel beautiful. This "imagined ugliness" is called body dysmorphic disorder. NET has been used successfully to assist patients in managing their anxiety through the surgical process. By releasing emotional blocks with NET, the patient heals and recovers faster and achieves a sense of wholeness, discovering her natural inner beauty. NET is effective in uncovering blocks which prevented the person from accepting her own inner beauty.

Jocelyn shares the example of a soon-to-be 30-year-old who came to Dr. Pendergrast's office crying and distraught about her appearance. She had been referred by her dermatologist to Dr. Pendergrast to take care of a severely infected cyst on her face which was not responding to antibiotics, incision, and drainage. An NET intervention was done after the infected cyst was treated. The NET session revealed a fear of intimacy with her boyfriend. After the release of past unconscious hidden emotions, she was transformed. She returned to the office the next week with an energetic, physical radiance, announcing her new wedding engagement. Evidently, her boyfriend proposed to her that weekend after the NET session. She was able to finally share her fears of intimacy, which brought them closer. The NET session had brought to her consciousness the reason she was having difficulty with their relationship and allowed her to reconcile with her boyfriend and to heal their relationship.

Jocelyn says, "With the permission of family members, I also use NET with neurologically intact elderly patients. I do muscle testing (kinesiology), asking the body questions. An extended arm will remain strong in the presence of truth; conversely, the same arm will weaken if a statement is false. The body never lies. Our bodies react to negative stressors by weakening and compromising our health. NET assists the body to become more congruent—mentally, emotionally, and physically. The body's energy can then flow naturally. NET is useful in the treatment of emotions trapped in the body and allowing the energy to flow naturally again. The body and subconscious mind do not forget unresolved wounds. In an effort to avoid the emotional pain from a traumatic event, the person suppresses the memory of the trauma. Rather than addressing the emotions, the feelings end up repressed and stored in the body's physiology, therefore blocking energy and inhibiting the natural healing response. This causes emotional and indirect physical disease."

Jocelyn reports working with a health-conscious elderly woman who wanted to lose weight because of arthritic knee pain. "She wanted to reduce weight the fast way using liposuction surgery. Being morbidly obese, she was considered a poor surgical candidate by Dr. Pendergrast. He told her that she needed to reduce her weight before he would consider liposuction. An NET session was recommended, which uncovered a traumatic event regarding her weight at age nine. Her teacher forced her to stand before the entire class and then proceeded to tell the class that she was an example of someone who was unhealthy and overweight. For the rest of her life, the woman's emotional energy was blocked by the memory of that horrific and humiliating event. The natural acceptance of herself and her body was inhibited by this memory. Through NET, she uncovered more events that reinforced these emotions of her poor self-image. She gained insight into her body's resistance to releasing the weight. Subsequently, she has reduced her weight and has become more successful in achieving better health, both physically and emotionally."

We [Jim and Linda] see distinct similarities between NET and an allergy treatment procedure called NAET, which stands for Nambudripad's Allergy Elimination Technique (see www.naet.com). As a staff nurse and NAET practitioner, Sue Huntley informs us, "Chinese medicine describes 12 major meridians; they are channels running deep in the tissues of the body, and through them flows an invisible energy that the Chinese call 'life force' (Henry and Henry 2004, p. 28). This energy which resides in and between our cells has been described by quantum physics. Think of each meridian as being a river of energy. Each one of these rivers of energy may be blocked by a 'dam', or allergy. If you have a dam in the river, water backs up, or in our case, energy backs up, creating illness. At the same time, downstream from the dam, not enough energy gets into the system creating the symptoms. The dam is removed through the rebalancing process, which involves massaging along the back of the body. A new message is sent to the brain and to every cell in the body. It informs the cells that the negative reaction is no longer necessary."

This new view of the universe as essentially flowing energy calls healthcare practitioners to be open to new paradigms. Many of these newer modalities offer aging adults opportunities for making choices, reviewing one's life, and no longer enduring past trauma and abuse. The competent practitioner must be aware of all choices in health care, including more traditional interventions, and know which modality is best for the patient. Jocelyn states, "I define a healthy person as one who is thoroughly alive, who can look back and know that they have done the best they could, considering life's circumstances. Such a person displays a certain level of resiliency, knowing that they encountered and overcame obstacles, gleaning a lesson of living from their tough times that can be passed on to others. Who they are and what they stood for over time makes a significant difference."

Caring for the elderly person with dementia and depression can be a challenge. Family members and professionals can promote meaningful and healthy aging. Jocelyn ends by saying, "Help them to keep their minds active by encouraging them to pursue hobbies and interests they enjoy. Keep your messages to them simple and concrete. Short instructions and sustained coaching are essential. Give them simple tasks followed by generous praise and rewards. Be patient, because directions may need to be repeated several times. It is the nature of dementia to change over time. On some days in the early stages, people with dementia may seem perfectly fine, while the later stages may bring unexpected abrupt moments of frustration and agitation. Caregivers must be careful not to project their frustration onto an elder. Without support for the primary caregiver, this potentially can lead to elder abuse. It is vital to empower the caregiver's sense of self-esteem and provide moments of rest and respite. Above all, caregivers need to see the big picture and not lose themselves within the caretaking process. Self-care is vital for life rejuvenation and is critical for feeling truly alive."

References

Childs-Gowell, E. 1992. *Good Grief Rituals.* Barrytown, New York: Station Hill Press.

Henry, L. & J. Henry. 2004. *The Soul of the Caring Nurse.* Silver Spring, MD: Nursesbooks.org.

Inouye, S.K., S.T. Bogardus, P.A. Charpentier, L. Leo-Summers, D. Acampora, T.F. Holford, & L.M. Cooney. 1999a. A multicomponent intervention to prevent delirium in hospitalized older patients. *New England Journal of Medicine* 340: 669–76.

Inouye, S.K., M.J. Schlesinger, & T.J. Lydon. 1999b. Delirium: a symptom of how hospital care is failing older persons and a window to improve quality of hospital care. *American Journal of Medicine* 106:565–73.

Inouye, S.K., S.T. Bogardus, D.I. Baker, L. Leo-Summers, & L.M. Cooney, et al. 2000. The Hospital Elder Life Program: A model of care to prevent cognitive and functional decline in hospitalized older patients. *Journal American Geriatric Society* 48:1697–1706.

Karnes, B. 2001. *Gone From My Sight—A Dying Experience.* Depoe Bay, OR: Barbara Karnes Books.

Leslie, D.L., Y. Zhang, S.T. Bogardus, T.F. Holford, L. Leo-Summers, & S.K. Inouye. 2005. Consequences of preventing delirium in hospitalized older adults on nursing home costs. *Journal American Geriatric Society* 53:405-9.

Rizzo, J.A., S.T. Bogardus, L. Leo-Summers, C.S. Williams, D. Acampora, & S.K. Inouye. 2001. Multicomponent targeted intervention to prevent delirium in hospitalized older patients: What is the economic value? *Medical Care* 39:740–52.

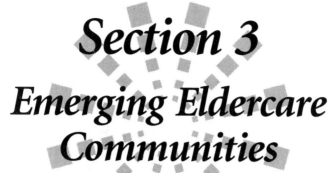

Section 3
Emerging Eldercare Communities

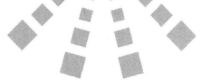

"*The longer I live, the more beautiful life becomes.*"
—Frank Lloyd Wright
(1869–1959)

In This Section . . . Transformational Eldercare communities are emerging throughout the United States and internationally. Eden Alternative™ leads the way and serves as a new model for a number of more traditional long-term care facilities. Some organizations innovate by constructing new small, home-like buildings built within small community settings. Aging in community and aging in place are emerging concepts of care.

Living life in the Garden of Eden: Sherbrooke Community Centre

Suellen Beatty, MScN, MSM

P eople need the opportunity to live until they die," believes Sherbrooke Community Centre CEO Suellen Beatty. That premise is the foundation of the Centre, which functions more like a small town than a long-term care facility. For many residents, it becomes almost like their entire world, so staff consciously works at creating community. Located in Saskatoon, Saskatchewan, Sherbrooke is a registered Eden Alternative™ home and represents a powerful model for improving the quality of life of elders. Rather than a program, Sherbrooke seeks to embody a total philosophy that Eden Alternative™ founder Bill Thomas, MD, describes as overcoming the three plagues of nursing homes: loneliness, helplessness, and boredom. While necessary, medical treatment alone fails to support quality of life and needs to be the servant and not the master of care.

"The best vehicle for creating community obviously becomes our staff," Suellen insists. "Our people invest so much more than what is written in their job descriptions. In a community of relationships, we encourage our staff to bring their whole personhood to work. I remember being taught in nursing school to leave your personality in the trunk of your car in the parking lot. But imagine that you are an elder living in a nursing home, cut off from the outside world. Each day you become exposed to staff members who raise their kids, go to the movies, and wear new fashions. The entire world is available to residents if our staff is willing to share their lives. So, what we do here is more like life care then health care. Obviously we must maintain some boundaries, but we promote bringing your life and your family to work with you. And, I must tell you that we have very few problems with boundaries."

Suellen entered health care by way of public health nursing in Saskatchewan, Canada. However, after a few years her passion began to fade, so she began working in a hospital in neonatal intensive care, pediatrics, and rehabilitation. She also taught at a nursing school, helping students deal with health situations that were very complex and counseling them that people were more than the piece of the puzzle that the nurse may be dealing with at the time.

Suellen maintains a great enthusiasm for learning and was especially impassioned by a two-week course in gerontology. "Coming out of my undergraduate program and working in a large university hospital, I had no idea that gerontology was even a specialty," she informs us. "There existed a body of knowledge and it seemed as though no one was sharing it, so I decided to go for a master's degree in gerontology, including the design of physical environments for people who are physically challenged. I was deeply drawn to the work of Florence Nightingale, who also placed great emphasis upon environmental issues. She believed that people's spirits were important and that they needed fresh air and sunshine."

Knowing her background in gerontology and the environment, in 1986 a group of people in Saskatoon invited her to work on the building of a new special-care home. At the time, a position of Director of Nursing was available; Suellen applied for it and was hired. Today, Suellen is the CEO, and they are beginning another building project. "I love this place and the people with whom I work," she states enthusiastically. " It's kept me interested because of the huge opportunity to learn. We provide services to 270 residents and to more than 100 people from the greater community who join us on a daily basis. The latter group enjoys the companionship, a hot meal, and some of the physical, occupational, and spiritual therapies. In addition, we have activities and clubs that just spring up around people's interests, like our wine-making club that produces wine used during many of our special occasions. We have about 150 people who have their own garden boxes accessible via wheelchairs. We even have our own radio station where people broadcast from within the facility."

Suellen states that Sherbrooke minimizes the establishment of formal programs. "Often these programs do not serve people well because they don't emanate from a philosophical base. We have a set of principles that shape our activities. I believe that if people understand the principles you don't need a whole lot of rules. For example, our first principle undergirds individuality: every elder is seen as an individual person without any stereotyping. Formal programs sometimes fail to support this principle because they often have to do with group activities. Rather, we attempt to connect with each individual. Our staff becomes involved in permanent relationships with the people for whom they provide care. We incorporate many healing modalities such as reminiscence, massage, and music therapies; but first we try to meet the needs of the individual.

"However, the program is essentially about *life*. It seems arrogant to program another person's life, which is what quite often happens in institutions. We envision Sherbrooke not as an institution but as the best place to live and the best place to work. We speak about this all of the time, about what this looks and feels like. We believe that if we care for the staff and they care for each other, then our clients will be well served. It's all about relationships, acknowledging that everyone has needs to be met. Therefore, staff receives as much worthy interest as the elders."

Suellen's vision for Sherbrooke includes even being the best place to die. Dying represents the last stage of living, all part of the same process. According to Suellen, the staff remains intimately involved in the dying process, making certain that people don't die alone. Almost all of the funerals are conducted on-site and candlelight ceremonies are held, giving people the opportunity to remember and celebrate the life of someone who has died.

In addition to the original building, the Sherbrooke facilities include 11 houses arranged in two villages called the Kinsmen and Veterans Villages. The village design is unique in relation to most special-care homes, states Suellen. Each fully equipped house has nine to ten residents and is attached to the rest of the facility by an internal street. "It's like having houses on any residential street, except that the street is internal and protected from the elements," she explains. "The houses are adaptable to the specialized needs of most groups of people including children, the disabled and frail elders, and a variety of cultures and groups with special functional needs such as those who suffer from Alzheimer's disease. Each of the 11 houses has at least one pet, including dogs, cats, rabbits, and birds. Not only do the pets help with loneliness and boredom, but they are a drawing card for children who wish to visit or volunteer."

The houses lend themselves to the formation of a more family-like group. Caregivers are called Daily Living Assistants (DLA), a title coined by the staff themselves. Multiskilled in running all aspects of running the household, the staff cooks meals, administers medications, and maintains an infection-free environment. Registered Nurses work in a model similar to home care, with the exception of not having to travel to see their clients.

The commitment to care and community radiates in these houses. Staff people share their lives with the residents and are welcome to bring their children to participate in the life of the house, especially on holidays. Residents love this sharing of family, which supports the commitment to alleviating loneliness. Because the DLA knows his or her residents intimately, meals can be customized to particular tastes. Suellen maintains, "Because they find themselves treated as individuals, people in the houses thrive more so than in traditional facilities."

Prior to constructing the villages, Suellen conducted focus groups with those who might be future clients. She found that most of them dreaded the prospect of becoming institutionalized in a traditional long-term care facility. She asked them to describe an ideal living arrangement when the time came that they could no longer fend for themselves. "They told us what they wanted and we built it," she recounts with pride. "It was that simple. The hard part involved convincing the healthcare providers and the government that this approach would work. However, we overcame the obstacles. Today people visit us from all over the world to learn more about this model."

Built in 1993, Sherbrooke continues to utilize their more traditional building. Because of regulations, it was the only alternative available to them at the time. However, groups of 20 residents, each with a private room, share common areas and are structured into "neighborhoods," which helps to create communities whereby elders continue the process of aging holistically and sharing their wisdom.

With respect to traditional long-term care facilities, Suellen informs us that people often enter them with a sense of dread. "People are very vulnerable at this stage of their lives, so they tend to conform to the rules and routines of the facility. This suppresses individual uniqueness, and after a period of time they become 'institutionalized.' It's not normal to be physically moved in with a large group of people and to have to adapt to the routines of healthcare professionals. As a nurse, I don't ever remember being trained to run somebody's life. However, this approach emanates from the cultural climate of many institutions. For this reason, we need smaller housing where you can more easily be yourself. Even in our more traditional building, we work to create smaller communities of people where everyone knows your name. We seek to create and support a culture where elders can be living libraries of knowledge and experience. Sherbrooke's mission is to provide an environment where residents can live full and abundant lives. This approach of being resident directed as opposed to resident centered means that we take direction from the residents rather than deciding what is in their best interests. It means that we serve as much as possible and try not to make decisions for the residents that we think are correct. Residents live by their own values, not by those imposed by the caregivers. People are so much more than the sum total of their parts, but somehow that gets lost in the current medical model."

Suellen supports the concepts outlined in gerotranscendence in the sense that she sees people arriving at the point where they don't have to understand everything. "A certain comfort arises when you can simply accept mystery and enjoy being in its presence," she reflects. "We are on a journey where our minds have been closed to so many of life's mysteries. However, the world seems to be unfolding before our eyes and manifesting itself in such healing modalities as acupuncture, Healing Touch, music therapy, and massage. We find ourselves attempting to figure out the underlying dynamics of why and how these work. It is a privilege to gain even a little insight and understanding."

Klein Center—Long-Term Life Enhancement

Amy Leilani Vandiver, Life Enhancement Coordinator

As the Life Enhancement Coordinator at the Great River Health System's Klein Center in West Burlington, Iowa, Amy Leilani Vandiver admits that her title is unusual. "Not only am I responsible for directing activities for our residents, but I also provide staff education and training," she explains. "So, this title really fits what I do." The Center, which became a certified Eden Alternative™ facility in 2005, cares for about 120 long-term residents.

Amy's love of working with elders began as a volunteer clown in a nursing home during her college days. "I loved it," she exclaims, "and one summer I worked at the home as an activities assistant." Her role consists of more than directing activities for the elderly. Her challenge also involves helping people to find continuing meaning and purpose in their lives. "It is important to assume that everyone has an inherent life purpose, even those elders who are somewhat restricted. We conduct a thorough social history of interests and abilities, encouraging residents to help their peers and give back to their families. We have started creating a scrapbook for each resident with pictures and a journal to which we will add pages occasionally. When possible, we also speak with the elder's family about her/his life journey.

"For example, one of our residents is Edna who is a wonderful artist and whose work is exhibited in our display cabinet. She serves others by helping others expand their art skills. In fact, she is currently teaching me to work with oil paints. So, our helping relationship is reciprocal."

As a part of the Great River Health System, The Klein Center frequently admits residents who have been hospital patients. The hospital developed an award-winning Living History Program as a way of learning more about the lives of older patients, particularly those who have been admitted multiple times. Storywriters, who are trained employees from various hospital departments, interview selected patients and write their life stories, which are then placed at the beginning of their patient-care charts. Caregivers are required to read them. The information can be used to establish connections between patients and employees. The storywriters also create a quick reference poster featuring a bridge that is then placed in patient rooms. When elders are later transferred to the Center, they bring with them information about their lives as depicted on the bridge. Words like "mother" or "musician" are placed across the span of the bridge. The support beams include biographical data such as place of birth, parents, and the like. The support cables include the names of children, grandchildren, and anyone else who provides support. The clouds above the bridge depict hobbies and activities that bring them pleasure. The bridge posters help staff members to connect immediately in a personal way with the new residents. Many of the hospital and Klein Center staff members receive training as storywriters. They also train volunteers how to read the bridges and to ask open-ended questions to solicit stories.

The impetus to become an Eden Alternative™ facility followed attending an introductory workshop. Professionally, founder Dr. Bill Thomas inspires Amy with his vision for changing eldercare. She considers him to be one of her greatest heroes and, in particular, has found his book, *Learning From Hannah: Secrets From a Life Worth Living*, particularly inspiring (Thomas 1999).

Amy believes that every facility, as good as it may be, has room for improvement. The Center and the Medical Center have been part of a customer service training program developed by Ron Willingham, entitled, *Hey, I'm the Customer* (Willingham 2003). "The emphasis on customer service really has impacted the way staff perceives patients and residents, making it much easier to becoming an Eden facility," Amy informs us. "The Eden organization conducted a 'soil warm test' of staff satisfaction. They told us our 'soil' was among the warmest they ever witnessed. In part, this results from treating every person, including staff and families, as customers."

Having gone through extensive training developed in the process of becoming an Eden facility, Amy believes that staff members better understand that loneliness, helplessness, and boredom represent severe issues in some eldercare facilities and use the same language in describing a resident's demeanor. "For example," explains Amy, "they might report that a person seems sad or bored. I mentioned Edna. When she first arrived, she became very irritable and demanding. Today she has become a wonderful person to be around. Another woman tended to sit in the back of the room during activities. We consciously look for such behaviors and seek to turn things around. As a result of Eden training and culture change, resident volunteers help with meetings, serve as greeters, and generally take charge of their home."

One of Eden's precepts in terms of making a facility seem more like home involves children. "My three-year-old daughter comes to work with me once each week," Amy reports with enthusiasm. "She plays games with residents, exercises with them and passes out candy. If you desire to transform eldercare, have a children's day care center near the facility. Also, we invite school kids to participate in activities and, at one time, had a Girl Scout group hold its meetings here. The residents participated in the program and actually earned badges. It doesn't cost anything to promote such intergenerational relationships."

To become an Eden Alternative™ facility, supervisors completed an initial ten-week course introducing them to ten basic principles (Thomas 2004) for a total of ten hours. The first two principles state the problem. The next three state the antidote for loneliness, helplessness, and boredom, focusing upon community and companionship. The final five principles tend to address more specific behaviors, where participants engage in training exercises. Supervisors then took an additional seven-week course with all of the staff for an additional eight hours. The supervisors complete a total of 18 hours of training, while staff go through eight hours of training. In addition, two CNAs, one LPN (licensed practical nurse), and a nutrition service worker went through all 18 hours.

Amy describes one training activity, which involves staff members writing ten words that people believe best describe them. Next, they write down ten words they believe that others would use to describe them. Then Amy places a sticker on everyone's forehead with words like, "I am hard of hearing," "I speak another language," "I am invisible," or "Treat me like a child," representing different labels and elder stereotypes. After everyone has their tags on, they start a conversation on sports, politics, etc., and participants then treat each other according to the label. The point of the exercise is to help people become more sensitive to how an older adult might describe him/herself, how families may respond, and how general cultural stereotypes impact them.

Not surprisingly, the Center enjoys a high employee retention rate. One of Eden Alternative's™ golden rules is that how management treats staff members is how staff treats residents. "Some of our staff came from other facilities so, in contrast, they see how an environment can be different," Amy underscores. "We stress teamwork in bimonthly departmental staff meetings, and there is an Excel Committee that periodically selects and honors employees exhibiting outstanding performance. We include residents in our activities. They often organize bridal and baby showers for the staff."

According to Amy, attention is given to the residents' spiritual needs. Chapel services are conducted on Tuesdays as well as Sunday afternoon devotions, led by a variety of area ministers. In addition, the residents who are Catholic gather to watch Mass on television, and a lay minister brings communion so they can participate at the same time as those on TV.

Finances are always of concern in most organizations providing long-term care. Amy acknowledges that the Klein Center is lucky in that it enjoys a trust fund that helps with the upkeep of the building and provides additional money for staff and services. They also receive funds from private paying residents and from Medicare and Medicaid. In addition, one factor of their Title 19 reimbursement is based on resident satisfaction. If resident satisfaction scores are higher than the state average, facilities receive a higher rate. The link between satisfaction and reimbursement is an Iowa State incentive. Amy reports that resident satisfaction always reaches such high levels that they receive a higher rate.

Amy believes passionately in her work. "We need to change current perceptions about aging. Elders should be honored for having lived through so many life events and circumstances," she states firmly.

TigerPlace

Marilyn Rantz, PhD, RN, FAAN

The very topic of moving into a nursing home often engenders a negative response, according to University of Missouri (MU) Sinclair School of Nursing professor, Marilyn Rantz. In the introduction to her book, *The New Nursing Homes*, she reports that "lack of privacy, bad smells, poor food, inadequate staff, separation from friends and family and an unpleasant environment are some of the things that pop into people's minds" (Rantz, Popejoy, & Zwygart-Stauffacher 2001, Intro., p. 1). According to Marilyn, however, today's "new" nursing homes are defying such stereotypes and are moving away from the institutional, hospital-like settings of the past. They offer more homelike, personalized care where staff members are more visible and attentive, family members are more involved, and facilities are cleaner and friendlier.

Having spent a significant amount of her career assessing nursing homes, Marilyn believes that the majority of them provide good care. "Even though you might have heard some reports and exposés to the contrary, most nursing homes hire people who are attempting to do a good job," she reports. "My advice to consumers when looking for a facility is to vote with your feet. When the care is substandard, as a consumer of care, you can't fix the problems by your presence. Obviously I advise people to find a good facility in the beginning, but always know that you can move loved ones."

In addition to her work as a professor, Marilyn serves as the director of TigerPlace, an exciting aging-in-place concept in community living developed through the collaboration of the MU Sinclair School of Nursing and Americare of Sikeston, Missouri (www.tigerplace.net). Because it falls out of the norm of a traditional living facility or nursing home, it was necessary to pass two rounds of state legislation in order to gain approval for the project. "In an assisted living facility when you need more care, you must move to the nursing home. At TigerPlace," notes Marilyn, "the vast majority of our clients remain in their apartments until they die." The name "Tiger" was selected because it is the name of the University of Missouri mascot.

TigerPlace is one of four pilot sites. "We were able to get legislation passed in Missouri allowing us to work around traditional regulations," Marilyn explains. "Residents at TigerPlace move in and receive services as needed with a home health model of care delivery. Although TigerPlace provides a basic package for all of its residents, including meals, people receive services based upon their needs. A wellness center is staffed by School of Nursing home health agency and offers a number of health promotion services such as exercise classes. Residents also enjoy access to a nurse on-call around the clock."

Each person or couple lives in one of 33 private apartments. "Not having to worry about becoming so frail that they would need to move helps people feel more secure and in control," Marilyn maintains. "TigerPlace does not look like a traditional nursing home. After consulting with a veterinary medicine clinic, the apartments were designed to be pet friendly, and there are walkways conducive to walking pets.

"Although costs are in line with the overall market rate for assisted living facilities, TigerPlace is a private-pay facility. Since the facility meets the code requirements for a nursing home and as a licensed intermediate care facility, costs can be covered by long-term care insurance. Hopefully, when enough outcome measures are established, we can convince the state that this works as a viable long-term care option eligible for coverage, including Medicaid." Marilyn believes that if the cost savings are such that people stay healthier longer, the model may be expanded.

The program involves students from various disciplines at the University, as well as faculty members who are involved in research projects. One such program is the Quality Improvement Program for Missouri (QIPMO), a joint project of the MU Sinclair School of Nursing and the Missouri Department of Health and Senior Services (DHSS). It is dedicated to helping facility staff develop quality improvement programs with actions that ultimately improve the quality of care in Missouri's nursing homes.

In another research project, after ten years of measuring the quality of care in nursing homes, an instrument was developed which included 30 targeted items to observe by walking through a nursing home (Rantz, Zwygart-Stauffacher, & Flesner 2005). Marilyn's hope is that consumers, other researchers, and nursing home regulators will adopt this instrument so they can benefit from targeting their observations and quickly judge quality of care. On the team's Web site, www.nursinghomehelp.org, there are numerous resources available:

- The *Consumers' Guide to Quality Care* offers advice for families searching for quality nursing home care.
- The *Providers' Guide to Quality Care* includes a case study and sample care plans clarifying many aspects of the Resident Assessment Instrument (RAI) and Minimum Data Set (MDS).
- The *Observable Indicators of Nursing Home Care (OIQ) Instrument* is a list of questions and ratings designed to measure the multidimensional concept of quality in nursing homes.

In a "new nursing home," residents are the center of concern. In her book, *Person-Centered Care*, Marilyn describes an Eden Alternative™ facility in Bethany, Missouri (Rantz & Flesner 2004). She commends the concept because it really puts residents at the center. Unless something is immoral or illegal, the Bethany facility's philosophy stipulates meeting their residents' requests. During the admitting process, people are asked to articulate what they wanted to accomplish at this stage of their lives, and the staff makes every effort to work with them collaboratively to make it happen.

"In the person-centered arena where I work, it becomes vital that people find and pursue meaning in their lives," Marilyn reports. "Purpose integrated with exercise and activity often leads to a healthier and longer life." For example, Dr. David Snowdon studied the abilities of a large number of nuns while living and their brains after they died, searching for signs related to dementia and other diseases (Snowdon 2001). He found that many were essentially asymptomatic because of their level of activity and engagement. In particular, learning at any age tends to be a health-promoting behavior, i.e., "Use it or lose it."

According to Marilyn, one of the most prevalent problems for elders is related to medications, a concern also noted by others in this book. Having multiple doctors who may not always be aware of the array of medications their patients are receiving can lead to medication mismanagement. Being aware of every drug an elder is taking, prescription and over-the-counter (OTC), is important for caregivers. Our research indicates that many physicians now are asking their patients to list all medications being taken, and an increasing number request that people bring in every medication including OTC drugs. Two other challenges for elders are eating a balanced nutritious diet and maintaining or regaining mobility. "Staying mobile is the key to aging well. Strength training with an active exercise program is vital to being able to do the things you want to be able to do and feeling good about your life," Marilyn affirms.

Additionally, Marilyn emphasizes the importance of having an understanding about some of the fundamental philosophies about aging. "Many stereotypes in this country work against healthy aging, such as the belief that everyone gets sick or experiences some degree of confusion linked to dementia," she says. "Not everyone gets Alzheimer's, and these stereotypes simply are not true relative to normal aging. Normal aging is not about losing function." She also underscores the importance of not just relating to older adults at the clinical level. "Connecting with people at a very real, personal level is essential. When we only relate to their problems clinically, nurses miss the important things that will really help them and motivate them to do things that will help them function and enjoy life."

KENDAL AT ITHACA

Dale R. Corson, Ph.D., and Maria Giampaolo, BS, CRT

D ale Corson's record is impressive. As the president of Cornell University from 1969 to 1977, Dale played an important role in bringing the university to stability during the Vietnam War student activism period, the civil rights disruptions, and the economic recession of the 1970s. A physicist, he discovered astatine, element 85 in the periodic table of elements, helped perfect the use of airborne radar during World War II, and led the establishment of the Sandia National Laboratory in New Mexico immediately following World War II.

Ninety-one at the time of the interview, Dale agrees with his wife in believing that his biggest legacy may well be his pivotal role in the development of Kendal at Ithaca. He was instrumental in making the retirement community possible, working with the developer, the architect, and the contractor to acquire the land and secure the financing as well as solving many other problems associated with the development. "Kendal enjoys a reputation for its intellectual and stimulating atmosphere," Dale reports with pride. "People don't come here to sit around and decay. The community's activities are formulated and coordinated by a large number of residents' committees. My particular focus is with the Art Display Committee, which manages an art gallery in one hallway in the building. All of the art is by local Ithaca artists, alternating between paintings and photography, displayed in rotating three-month exhibits. Biannually we also sponsor a craft exhibit." A semiprofessional photographer, Dale notes modestly that about 50 of his photographs, mostly of nature, hang permanently in the facility.

Even while president of the university, Dale began working on the idea of having a retirement community nearby. As the chairman of the organizing group, Dale dedicated nearly six years of his life to the development of the community, which opened in late 1995. After visiting a number of facilities around the country, it was decided that the Kendal Corporation seemed to be the best developer to meet their criteria. Kendal at Ithaca is associated with the Kendal Corporation, a not-for-profit organization based in Kennett Square, Pennsylvania, dedicated to building a system of retirement communities in accordance with the principles of the Quakers (Religious Society of Friends).

Most of their facilities are located near colleges and universities, providing their residents with a wide range of intellectual and cultural opportunities pioneering the spirit of quality of life and learning. Nationally recognized as a leader in serving older people, Kendal's approach is based on the philosophy that retirement and growing older can bring new opportunities for growth and development.

Since its opening, Kendal at Ithaca has attracted Cornell alumni, as well as others, from around the country. Because a large number of renowned physicists live at Kendal, residents boast that Cornell University in Ithaca has the second best physics department in the country, surpassed only by Kendal.

Kendal at Ithaca is one of a number of lifelong learning retirement communities that are being developed nationally near colleges and universities, as universities and developers realize the appeal of a college campus and the numerous resources the schools bring to retirees. The retirement community offers clustered cottages or apartments in varying sizes with residential services, including one meal a day. Among the health services available are primary health care with complete annual physical exams, routine health screening, and wellness programs. A nurse-practitioner is on-site, and several physicians see their patients on-site. Residential services include assisted living and skilled nursing care units. Dental care is available on a part-time basis.

The community also features a day care center for preschool-age children that incorporates intergenerational programming, and the Community Center facilities house dining and activity areas as well as a bank and beauty shop.

Dale concludes that one of the most important challenges of the aging process is to keep active intellectually. "I've generally done this myself," he reports. "I've lost my ability to perform mathematics relative to my younger years. However, after I retired in 1979, I spent most of the next 15 years working in Washington for the National Academy of Sciences, National Academy of Engineering, the National Science Foundation, World Bank, and the White House (working through the President's Science Advisor)."

During his retirement, Dale has been involved with a number of interesting projects, including serving as the chairman of an international advisory committee on a several-hundred-million dollar World Bank loan to China for the purpose of upgrading their university science and engineering programs.

Dale's advice to the baby boomers who are approaching their older years is to find a continuing purpose for their lives and to keep active. "There are many retirement communities built on golf courses. That's not my idea of keeping active mentally," he says emphatically. "I used to play golf regularly—that is, once a year. Fortunately, today there are many communities like Kendal, continuing care facilities that are oriented toward life enhancement rather than diminishment."

As a Certified Recreational Therapist working in the adult home and skilled nursing facilities of Kendal, Maria Giampaolo helps people engage in caring, meaningful life activities as they move toward the end of their lives. It is her passion.

The Kendal residents reflect a variety of physical situations, from those needing more assistance because of general aging to people recovering from strokes or who have dementia. The challenge is adapting a variety of activities so that all individuals can participate in them.

"Of course, exercising is quite important to residents," Maria underscores. "They participate in a variety of adaptive exercise opportunities such as T'ai Chi, walking, and strength development through the use of weights. Kendal is somewhat unique in that the environment reflects the need for intellectual stimulus, so we involve residents in a number of discussion groups. For example, in the health center you will see a bulletin board display about 'Where in the world have you been?' Our residents are well traveled, so we will pick different countries, conduct research, and share stories about their experiences. They become very involved and engaged in the topic."

Maria supports the belief that reminiscence therapy is extremely important for elders. "Just talking about significant, past, historical events is healing—the Great Depression, what college was like and so on. We have a display in one of our activity rooms called 'Remember when.' We took old products like Burma Shave and encouraged people to recall and share memories. You can learn so much by listening to these stories."

We also highly recommend the use of OH Cards. OH Cards are sets of 88 picture cards and 88 word cards. You place the picture card on top of the word card and tell a story. The cards provoke sharing and insight, bringing to a conscious level many experiences in life. A total of 7,744 combinations are possible. The cards and instructions can be purchased from Eros Interactive Cards, 1-800-236-1683 or via their Web site at www.OH-cards.com.

In addition, the use of a PBS Home Video featuring Thomas Moore, entitled *Discovering Everyday Spirituality – Story,* can be very effective in promoting storytelling. It is divided into various segments, with Moore providing some background information followed by vignettes. Stop the video after each segment and involve the group in a discussion. For example, the first vignette is a mother describing to her little daughter the situation surrounding her birth. Group members would follow this by sharing stories regarding their earliest memories as a child. The video can be found at most public libraries, especially in larger communities. It may also be purchased via the Internet. Other videos in this series include *Place, Activity,* and *Rituals.*

Music therapy serves as a special source of engagement for the more frail Kendal residents. "We have residents who don't respond to verbal conversations, but if you turn on a particular kind of music, they are able to sing, remembering the words. We often see their facial expressions light up.

"Of course, we include art therapy in the activities, involving residents in meaningful art crafts that are small and simple. For example, at the moment we are making reminiscent-type quilts. The topic of each resident's quilt is 'Lessons of a life time.' Whatever lesson learned will be included in the quilt, becoming another creative way to preserve a person's legacy.

"Another quite interesting project involved having elders paint pictures of their hands," Maria continues. "People put their hand print on a square, finishing the phrase 'These are the hands that have. . . .' For example, someone might say, 'These are the hands that shook hands with FDR,' or 'These are the hands that engineered bridges.' All of the hand prints and explanations were gathered in the form of a collage for display in the hallway."

Sitting atop a hill outside Ithaca, Kendal is shaped in a way that supports attractive horticulture. Garden carts designed to accommodate an individual's physical limitations have been made by some of the residents in the woodworking shop. The Kendal community also enjoys a unique philosophy in that some of the residents want to make certain that no segregation occurs between the different levels of care. "One Kendal" is a volunteer group of residents dedicated to community-enhancement volunteering. An "Escort Group" helps residents in wheelchairs attend special events. "Comfort Watch" is a trained group of volunteers who sit with residents while they are dying, if and when family is unavailable or needs respite.

Celebrations occur after death as well, Maria informs us. "Often when a resident passes away, the family will schedule the memorial service at Kendal. In addition, residents might plant a tree in memory of a friend or give something to the Kendal community. At Thanksgiving, the community holds a remembrance service planned by the interfaith committee. As part of it, a rose is placed in a vase as a list of the names of residents who have passed away is read.

"When someone dies in the health center, we find it awkward to walk by the empty room. Therefore, we began a tradition whereby a flower and perhaps the person's picture are placed outside the door. Actually, this was initiated by staff members who were having a hard time grieving the person's loss.

"My biggest joy is in getting to know and to develop friendships with the residents, motivating them to participate in activities that bring meaning and enjoyment," Maria affirms, "I receive great pleasure in knowing that my work makes a difference to their quality of life."

ElderHealth Northwest—Aging in Community

Nora Gibson, MSW, Teresa Hernandez, CNA, and Donna Bergman, BA

Walking into Buchanan Place, we saw several people assisting with various everyday living tasks. One gentleman was helping to unload groceries that had just been delivered. Dorothy, who has dementia, was folding laundry. She smiled, looked up, and told us with obvious delight, "I love to do this!"

"Such a wonderful response to being able to do an ordinary task," says ElderHealth Northwest Executive Director Nora Gibson, enthusiastically. The overarching goal of ElderHealth is to enhance the quality of life for frail elders and those with chronic illnesses and disabilities. "We want to help frail adults to remain living in their own homes with their families whenever possible," she explains. "ElderHealth Northwest is really about community. We have adult day health centers, geriatric care management, in-home care, volunteer companionship, and most recently we have added two supported living homes as alternatives to skilled nursing and assisted living facilities" (www.elderhealth.org).

ElderHealth has been in the Seattle area for over 25 years and was among the first adult day health providers in the country. Today, they have multiple adult day health centers scattered throughout the Seattle area. Recognized nationally as an innovative leader in the field of adult day health care, the Robert Wood Johnson Foundation, the largest U.S. foundation devoted to health care, honors ElderHealth Northwest as a National Model Adult Day Center. The Brookdale Foundation also uses ElderHealth as a model for new adult day programs starting up across the country.

In addition to five adult day health centers, Nora oversees two residences and services for a total of between 600 and 700 people. Gaffney House, a beautiful home built in 1903 that is listed in the National Register of Historic Places, can accommodate up to 16 people and is private pay. Buchanan Place was built from the ground up and is nestled among homes in a quiet residential neighborhood next to one of the adult day centers and is able to accommodate 12 people. Only a discreet brass plaque identifies it.

As the Lead Resident Assistant at ElderHealth's Buchanan Place, Teresa Hernandez, CNA, does just about everything a person would do in managing a general household—cooking meals, cleaning, and making beds, as well as scheduling and participating in daily tasks and activities. She serves as a caregiver for 12 residents ranging from ages 67 to 100 years old.

Having worked in a more traditional nursing home with 80-plus residents for four years prior to joining ElderHealth, Teresa finds the contrast between her two experiences significant. "At Buchanan Place, there is much more one-on-one time, so we can determine what the residents like and need," she informs us. "In addition, almost all of our residents have visitors, whereas in the previous place where I worked, family members often ignored people. Just because a family places a parent or grandparent in a facility doesn't mean that they don't have to visit," she says emphatically.

"Our residents have more choices than in many other residential facilities," Teresa explains. "When I order food, for example, I ask them for input. Sometimes I must cook specific foods for an individual. In addition, they can determine their own daily schedule with respect to bathing and the like. Because each person has an individual room, they have their own space, which is important. We have a much homier and more comfortable environment, and our staff members do not wear uniforms.

"Many of our residents come to us from other facilities," Teresa reports. "Their families often inform us that their family members were not being cared for very well. But here, residents and family members alike may speak with any person they desire, including our director."

Having an adult day center next to the residence is a major advantage for people in terms of giving them a variety of activities and options, Teresa states. "One of our older residents often exclaims, 'Oh, I get to go to school,' and becomes quite excited about the prospect."

Teresa continues working within the environment because, as she says, "I simply enjoy it, and I view caring for these residents as though they were my grandparents. I ask myself how I would like my family elders to be treated. I function as if I were a guest in someone's home. In addition, there can be no doubt that the residents view Buchanan Place as their home. They have their own possessions in their own space, just like they were at home."

Most of the residents exhibit some stage of dementia in addition to frailty and physical disability. Almost half moved out of nursing homes into the setting, and all are considered "nursing home eligible," a criterion for their funding through the Washington State Medicaid-funded waiver program known as COPES (Community Options Program Entry System). For this group of frail elders, the goal is to provide the most pleasant experience possible, something we could envision for ourselves. Opened in 2004, it was built with a combination of funding sources, including government funds.

"Adult day centers have existed since the 1970s," notes Nora. "They take components of what services would be available if you moved into a nursing home and make them available in the community where you live. These centers include ongoing, supportive nursing, maintenance rehabilitation services for people with disabilities, social work, mental health care, exercise, various activities, and socialization, all of which can help elders remain in their homes for a much longer period. Currently we have about 20 staff members at the center adjacent to Buchanan Place."

Donna Bergman, BA, is one of them. As a case manager, Donna enjoys working with about 25 people on her caseload, although the center sees 50–90 people daily. She is the point person serving as their advocate, making certain that they have the care and resources they need. She also coordinates the development of quarterly care plans and communicates with physicians and other staff personnel.

Interestingly, Donna's college degree was in theater. "I took a year off from school to care for a sick family member and during that time reassessed my life's direction," she relates. "I decided that we only live once, so why not make it fun. So, I switched my education from nursing to theater, which was great."

Her mother had already been working in eldercare and suggested that she try it out as a way of making a living. "For some reason, it just worked for me and gave me great satisfaction," Donna reports. "Also, I found myself able to use my theater background. I began entertaining people in the adult day center and even organized a theater group. We had a drama therapy group that worked for more than two months on a Christmas pageant. Even people who are nonverbal could participate by doing something tactile such as putting on a beard."

An African-American, Donna believes that her race is an asset. "I think it is an asset because we have a lot of African-American elders who can connect somewhat better with me, often because I remind them of a grandchild or some other person in their past and so that helps reduce anxiety. My skin tone can actually be calming."

Again, our conversation with Donna reminds us of three forms of discrimination in our culture: racism, sexism, and ageism. Black, elderly females might find themselves exposed to all three being dumped on them. On the other hand, because of such life experiences, these women perhaps are among the wisest in our society. Donna agrees, saying, "They have a sense of kindness as well as an element of sheer strength. They can be both tough and wonderfully sweet."

Donna's work activities are broad in scope and in the near future will include art therapy. The underlying goal of all activities involves providing a safe zone for people to participate in community and to satisfy their need for routine and structure, Donna explains. "What we do enhances the general well-being of people. So many elders tend to be socially isolated because they have lost a lot of family and friends. The center provides a place where people feel wanted and appreciated."

For this very reason, Donna confirms the reality that staff working at the center cannot put on a mask and fake personal feelings and issues. "Personal anxiety and fears can be sensed by others," she underscores. "Somehow this energy crosses over to everyone else. We need to be honest and inform people when we are not having a very good day. Without dumping on clients, sometimes we will say, 'You are so wise, give me some advice,' which is a way of having a community discussion. Or, we need to communicate with fellow staff members to see if tasks can be switched around in order to get through the day. Staff members understand that everyone has a bad day, so they are always willing to help."

With its many challenges, we wondered what keeps Donna working in the eldercare environment. Hesitating, she reflects, "Sometimes I don't know; yet I have so much invested in this work and sense how great it is to be involved in a terrific agency. Then there are those wonderful small moments when someone speaks for the first time in months. Sometimes I feel selfish, like I am able to give back to people, if even in a small way, and enjoy myself in the process."

According to Donna, ElderHealth is sensitive to employee stress. "The agency also offers monthly paid time off (PTO), which for most of us translates to a paid mental health day. This is encouraged by my supervisor and team members, and while expensive, it is cheaper than dealing with a high turnover rate. Most of my peers came to ElderHealth from other nursing homes and report a huge difference in the work environment, especially in terms of lower staff/client ratios. And, here we have a strong sense of working as a team."

For the last several years, Nora has given considerable thought to the idea of taking these service-rich adult day centers and using them as neighborhood service hubs. "Several components could be added, such as home care as well as residential care," she explains. "In this manner, both staff and services could be shared. The residential, boarding home could take care of the very frail population with clinically challenging issues. On the home care side, employees would leave from the day center and work in people's homes. Reporting to the clinical staff, the ability to problem solve would be tremendous, spreading professionalism in areas typically not available. Keeping the radius of the service area small is important. Currently many home care agencies find themselves required to serve an entire county. With a day center hub, you could have centralized administration but decentralized residential care."

Admittedly, retaining staff members who have a passion for caring can be challenging. The intent at ElderHealth is to have staff cross-trained in various functions so they can be fairly paid and enjoy full benefits, which results in a low turnover rate, notes Nora. "Our staff works a 40-hour week that can consist of different jobs." Typically in the home care and boarding house environments, workers receive an hourly wage and do not enjoy benefits.

Each day health facility enjoys the services of an activity director. However, the entire staff also participates in events and projects. "One of my expectations is that the entire staff, including me, be involved with all aspects of care, such as helping people in the bathroom," Nora points out. "I strongly dislike hierarchies where the most difficult tasks, such as personal care, are assigned to people who are paid less. I call it 'role-blurring.' Obviously, the nurses have specific training and duties, but everyone knows how to deal with explicit challenges on the job, physical and otherwise."

Nora believes that the appropriate way to connect with people who enter the facilities is by ascertaining who they are and what they have to offer. This is especially true in a small group community model. Even in a day center where the numbers expand, it becomes easier to get to know personal stories because they remain outside a resident facility.

ElderHealth enjoys the support of volunteers through a program called Elder Friends. They recruit and train volunteers from the community, conduct background checks, and match them with elders who are isolated and living alone without support. The primary focus is upon building relationships and doing routine chores. Nora reports, "If I had a lot of money, I would greatly expand this program. Like hurricane-ravaged places such as New Orleans, unfortunately our community contains many thousands of elders who are isolated and invisible. It becomes vital that we develop a mechanism that would reach to out to those people who need someone to be a friend and to worry about them. When there is a significant event like a snowstorm, someone is available to check in with them. Elder Friends essentially costs very little. Currently, the core of our volunteers are younger people in their twenties and thirties with children, whose own parents are living independently and who desire to be of service to other elders. Another group that might be of assistance is the older baby boomers who are retiring, linking them to people in their eighties and beyond."

As a relatively new model, Nora plans to refine ElderHealth's integrated systems before expanding the concept. Within the next five years, Nora plans to look for creative financing options to build several more boarding homes like Buchanan Place in close proximity to adult day centers. Keeping residents in neighborhoods prevents having to move to an environment where everyone else is a frail elder. She states, "From the outside, you can't tell that Buchanan Place is a residence for elders. And, when they are taken to the nearby farmer's market, they actually pick vegetables to prepare for dinner that night. It is not the most efficient model, which would be to start a campus away from the community. That is where the ideal rubs against financial realties. However, through creative financing similar to programs of building low-income housing, it could be done. In addition, it may be possible to organize a kind of 'Habitat for Elder Humanity.'"

ElderHealth receives its funds from Medicaid, the Washington State Senior Services Act, the Respite Program, the Veterans Administration, and private pay. Unfortunately, the current payment rate for Medicaid has not changed for the past ten years. "In the State of Washington," Nora underscores, "we are working to get an increase. However, at least in the world of Medicaid, if we see huge cutbacks, the possibility for innovation will disappear."

We asked Nora to help us understand how their organization can survive, given such constraints. She underlines that management must really work hard at finding creative ways to work with the funds that are available. For example, with Buchanan Place, which is licensed as a boarding home, she applied for and received low-income housing funds from city and state agencies. It has no debt service because it is considered a low-income residence. Some of the residents also use the day center, so they add revenue to the entire system.

Nora believes that the momentum for significant, transformational eldercare will emerge when our culture realizes that its elders are walking libraries and human resources of great wisdom. As this message surfaces and gains greater acceptance, then great change will take place. She believes the Eden Alternative™ and Greenhouse models provide us with a wonderful vision of what the future could look like, moving frail eldercare away from being a combination of poor house and hospital.

ADULT FAMILY HOME SETTING

Lisa Jackson, CNA

Lisa Jackson's eyes shine when she talks about "my ladies." Lisa operates an adult family home where she cares for six women, all of whom are in varying stages of dementia or Alzheimer's disease. "Lilly is my oldest lady at 106, and I know she will be with us when she turns 107 next November."

Lisa provides the total care 24/7 with the help of one employee who comes in one day a week to give Lisa time away. She also stays with the women while Lisa takes someone to the doctor or during the time when those who are able go out to have their hair done and then to lunch. "We have so much fun when we go out," Lisa smiles. "I think it is important for the ladies to have different socialization experiences. We have a number of outings, including going to the fair each year. They really enjoy going out."

Lisa admits that being the sole caregiver 24/7 is unusual for most adult home operators. "Many owners buy the homes and then hire a staff. I want to be here because I like to know what is happening with my ladies," she explains. "When I am with them all of the time, I am aware of any subtle physical changes and can then alert their physician." More than once, she has helped to identify the early symptoms of congestive heart failure. "I also find that they change almost on a daily basis. For example, there are marked behavior changes when there is a full moon or if they have a urinary tract infection." Lisa's experiences support research that suggests that when physical and mental functions decline, other senses become more acute. "For example, for the few days around a full moon, Esther doesn't need her walker and seems to be able to walk as well as I can at this time."

According to Lisa, many of the ladies are taking numerous medications when they move into the home. "Medicine can sometimes be harmful, and because I am with them and know them, I've been able to help them eliminate the medications they no longer need. For example, Lois reduced her regime from 14 pills a day to only 6," she reports.

Lisa's conversation is peppered with stories about "her ladies," and she likes to bring out the photo albums filled with their pictures taken in a variety of settings in and around the home and during outings. She also keeps the pictures of every resident she has cared for on a bulletin board in the kitchen. "Once the ladies move in, they are here until they pass away. Annie and Callie were here for eight years, the longest amount of time I have had anyone. Annie's sister was the one of the first residents when my mother owned the home. When Annie came to visit, she told my mother that if she ever got sick, this is where she wanted to come. So, this is where her son brought her. She was a character," Lisa recalls laughing.

"I love all my ladies," she says warmly. "They are really like my grandmother. Although it is hard when someone you love dies," she acknowledges, "I feel like they are watching over me.

"The women have so many interesting stories to share. Lilly was born in 1899 at a time when there were no cars, TV, or other modern conveniences. Now, she is living into a third century. I wish we could capture all the things she has seen. I was making a bonnet in preparation for the pictures we were going to take for Thanksgiving cards we were making when Lilly saw me stitching the bonnet by hand. She looked up and said 'bonnet.' Of course, that's what she wore for many years."

Lisa believes that the warm, personal attention and care the ladies receive in the home setting adds quality and years to their lives. "When Beadie came here, she had stopped eating and drinking and she was close to renal failure. She was in the hospital and had to receive two pints of blood from stomach ulcers. I think her deterioration was from loneliness. She was by herself in a senior residence where she had her own little place and she was left by herself. I got her on the day she got out of the hospital because I had taken care of her sister. Soon she began to flourish, eating and drinking, and she returned to a higher functioning level. She had been on a lot of psychotropic drugs and multiple drugs that had aspirin in them. When she didn't eat or drink, they led to the ulcers. After she moved in, we were able to reduce the number of her medications by half."

As with Beadie and Annie, Lisa informs us, once a family sees the caring family atmosphere provided, it is not unusual to care for another member of the family who moves in when they need such care. "Too often, people in nursing homes are simply left alone," Lisa says sadly. "Unfortunately, sometimes there are caregivers in larger nursing homes who don't really care about the residents."

Lisa reports that each of the women has their own physician, and family members typically take them for medical appointments. "If that's not possible, then I will take them for their appointments," she explains. "We also have a visiting nurse who comes at least monthly. She is very helpful and we go over everything that is happening and all the various drugs people take. I know that I can call her at any time and she will be here."

The days are filled with activities. "I love to cook and bake, and although I don't want them to be close to the stove, I always ask them what they want to eat. Usually, they will say, 'Whatever you want to cook, we'll love it.' Often someone will fold clothes." In the summer, Lisa's yard is full of flowers, and the group enjoys sitting outside on the patio.

"The ladies enjoy particular TV shows and movies, especially *Little House on the Prairie, Matlock*, some of the game shows, and *Golden Girls*. The ladies love our neighbor's little girls," Lisa says pointing to pictures of one of the women holding a baby and feeding her. "The girls will bring a movie over and they will all sit watching and laughing together." At other times, Lisa reports, there are craft activities. "Beadie likes to color. For Halloween, Thanksgiving, and Christmas we took pictures of each lady wearing special holiday hats, which we pasted on the cards. They wrote something inside and then we mailed them to their families. I like to challenge them. Also, we have someone who plays accordion music here once a month."

Some of the women attend church periodically when driven by their families. "I tried to get someone in a Catholic church to pick up Esther to take her to church, but I couldn't find anyone. Because of the diverse religions represented, I can't really coordinate in-home services. We do have a couple of different pastors visit their members."

Lisa began her career working with elders in a nursing home at the age of 15, where she remained for 13 years. Although she later worked in other retail businesses and managed a physician's front office, she returned to caring for older adults when she agreed to take over the adult home run by her mother when she retired. "Adult family homes must meet rigid standards, are licensed by the state, and are inspected annually," Lisa reports. "I am a Certified Nurses Assistant (CNA) and am required to keep up my class work each year. Although there is an Adult Family Home Association, I don't belong because I don't want to be away attending meetings."

Making the decision to place a family member in an alternative living situation is admittedly difficult, Lisa agrees. "When someone is considering an adult family home, I advise them to personally inspect it for cleanliness and whether it smells. You can tell if the residents appear happy or whether they are isolated and stay in their rooms. The ladies here don't usually go to their rooms until it's time to go to bed. I also suggest families check whether the owner of the house is there or who the staff members are." Although not all adult family homes accept Medicare and Medicaid, Lisa accepts both.

While Lisa admits that there is stress in managing the home continuously, she loves her work. "I can't get sick," she laughs. "It's worth it during the times when the ladies are lucid and express their love and appreciation."

References

Rantz, M. & M. Flesner. 2004. *Person-Centered Care*. Silver Spring, MD: Nursesbooks.org.

Rantz, M., L. Popejoy, & M. Zwygart-Stauffacher. 2001. *The New Nursing Homes*. Minneapolis: Fairview Press.

Rantz M., M. Zwygart-Stauffacher, & M. Flesner. 2005. Advances in measuring quality of care in nursing homes: a new tool for providers, consumers, regulators, and researchers. *Journal of Nursing Care Quality* 20(4):293-6.

Snowdon, D. 2001. *Aging With Grace.* New York: Bantam.

Thomas, W. 1999. *Learning From Hannah: Secrets for a Life Worth Living.* Acton, MA: VanderWyk & Burnham.

Thomas, W. 2004. *What Are Old People For?* Acton, MA: VanderWyk & Burnham.

Willingham, R. 2003. *Hey, I'm the Customer.* Upper Saddle River, NJ: Prentice Hall.

Section 4
Higher Education and In-House Training Programs

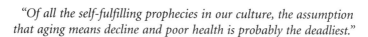

"Of all the self-fulfilling prophecies in our culture, the assumption that aging means decline and poor health is probably the deadliest."

—Marilyn Ferguson, *The Aquarian Conspiracy*

In This Section . . . A growing number of healthcare organizations are beginning to recognize older adults as their core business. Roughly 50% of all hospital beds are filled by people 65 or older. Yet, nursing schools are only now beginning to appreciate the importance of geriatric content in their curricula. The John A. Hartford Foundation supports many of the educational innovations taking place today.

BUILDING GERIATRIC NURSING CAPACITY

Patricia D. Franklin, MSN, RN

The coming crisis of dwindling numbers of nurses coupled with the onslaught of an aging population may be likened to a perfect storm, according to Patricia D. Franklin, Program Manager, The American Academy of Nursing Coordinating Center. "The nursing workforce is decreasing. We are reaching a critical period where the number of graduating nurses and the number entering the workforce are outpaced by those retiring and leaving. At the same time, we are faced with the reality of the enormous increase in the aging population. When these two collide, it could be catastrophic, definitely a health crisis for our country," she explains. "We certainly want to avert that situation.

"Caring for the elderly is a field that we are still discovering," claims Patty. She affirms the importance of providing nurses with a high level of preparation and education to meet the needs of the growing elderly population. "In the seventies, it was not uncommon to use long-term care facilities for first year nursing students to begin learning their basic clinical practice skills," she recalls. In retrospect, she believes that practice to be a disservice, not only to the residents but also to the nursing students who were not equipped to care for that population. "We know that the fragile skin of the elderly requires specific care, different from that of young adult patients, for example. Additionally, the health status of the elderly is very complex, and they often face multiple issues. We need caregivers who are well informed and understand how to differentiate dementia from confusion as a result of medication. However, long-term care facilities can be wonderful experiences when the students' knowledge and skills are well matched with the level of care required by the resident."

According to Patty, the number of community sites that provide care and services to elders also can be excellent placement opportunities for nursing students. "The Hartford Centers of Geriatric Nursing Excellence and the Hartford Nursing School Geriatric Investment schools of nursing look for available clinical sites and where to position students so that appropriate clinical experiences are provided for the students' skill levels and their experience will be gratifying. Nursing students can enter the eldercare system at all different levels of their education, but it is essential to match their level of skills with the needs of the elderly, from learning interviewing skills with elders in the community to complex clinical responsibilities with elderly patients in acute care settings."

Although there are some 670 universities offering nursing programs at the baccalaureate level, less than one-third have even one geriatric nursing faculty. However, Patty believes that there is a growing awareness of gerontology. "We can look to pediatrics and possibly other specialty areas where there is a defined, unique difference in those populations. Those in the field of pediatrics worked hard to have children recognized as not just little adults, but as having their own distinctive developmental, psychological, and physiological needs. Correspondingly, the field of geriatrics is growing too, and we are recognizing that the elderly are not just adults who have lived longer," explains Patty. "Their bodies are changing, and they too have unique psychological, social, and physiological needs. The field of geriatric nursing is growing, and with it is the need for developing evidence-based care rooted in that science, which must be translated and conveyed to the nursing workforce. Consequently, we need to have a cadre of nurse educators prepared in geriatric nursing, as well as conducting the research to build the science that provides a stronger foundation of evidence-based care."

According to Patty, there have been important and exciting developments in the arena of geriatric nursing. The Hartford Foundation Institute for Geriatric Nursing at New York University is the flagship geriatric nursing initiative funded by the John A. Hartford Foundation (JAHF), providing resources and information for nurses caring for geriatric patients. The Institute has expanded its scope to include programs for nurse educators and researchers and also reached out to the specialty nursing organizations.

"The Hartford Foundation recognizes that nurses are at the center of health care, especially in geriatrics," notes Patty. "JAHF is a philanthropic organization that now devotes all of its philanthropy and resources to improving care for the elderly. Beginning with the Hartford Institute in 1996, the JAHF then partnered with the American Academy of Nursing in 2000 to design a program that would build academic geriatric nursing capacity within schools of nursing by preparing the faculty to teach the emerging workforce, which will care for the growing elderly population.

"The Academy provides the Coordinating Center, which manages the JAHF funded nursing initiative, 'Building Academic Geriatric Nursing Capacity (BAGNC).' This program enjoyed the leadership of Dr. Claire M. Fagin as Program Director for the first five years. Beginning in July, 2005, Dr. Patricia Archbold assumed the role of Program Director. This exciting program provides scholarships for nurses entering or already enrolled in a PhD nursing program. The two-year scholarship program offers financial support as well as leadership-building activities. We sponsor an annual leadership conference as well as other leadership-enhancing activities," notes Patty. "In addition, the program offers a two-year fellowship for doctorally prepared nurse faculty to support their research in this field. While hopefully we are attracting the brightest and best and most committed and passionate nurses we can find, the program also focuses on developing leadership skills, which are essential to move the field toward a model of quality care for all elderly citizens."

To date, the program has supported 106 scholarships and fellowships. The full impact of this initiative will not be evident for a number of years; however, the graduating classes already demonstrate significant achievements in publishing in peer reviewed journals, attaining faculty appointments, and receiving funding for their research projects. The initial success of the first five years provided sufficient evidence to earn another five-year funded award by the John A. Hartford Foundation. Two additional partners have joined this initiative providing support to the scholars and awards: The Atlantic Philanthropies and The Mayday Fund.

The BAGNC programs include five Hartford Centers of Geriatric Nursing Excellence that are located at the University of California San Francisco (USCF), Oregon Health and Science University (OHSU), University of Arkansas Medical Sciences in Little Rock, University of Iowa, Iowa City, and the University of Pennsylvania in Philadelphia. "These Centers were funded by the John A. Hartford Foundation because they were recognized as schools of nursing with significant programs in geriatric nursing which, with investment, would further develop programs of geriatric nursing research, practice, education, and leadership in the field. A special issue of *Nursing Outlook* was to be published in early 2006, providing a cross-center report on the remarkable achievements conducted both within these centers and through joint endeavors.

"Almost 50% of our scholars and fellows attend these centers. The other 50% are located across the country. Since the program's inception in July 2000, 106 scholarships and fellowships were granted within 39 different universities in 24 states and DC, located from New York to Hawaii. We are committed to targeting states where we don't have any scholars at this time, to build capacity in those regions. It's not a passive program," emphasizes Patty. "It's a very active, strategic initiative with a nationwide impact.

"The John A. Hartford Foundation also invested in seven additional schools of nursing in 2002 that are just finishing their program. Funding was given to these seven schools of nursing to build their geriatric programs. The results are stunning. New curricula, Web-based and outreach programs, were created along with developing new clinical sites and clinical programs for teaching nurses geriatric health care. A number of these schools of nursing developed partnerships in their communities with long-term care and other facilities caring for the elderly, and The University of Minnesota held an international research summit. There is a tremendous momentum building as a result of these programs.

"The Academy's BAGNC program also partners with other Hartford-funded geriatric nursing programs including the Hartford Institute and those coordinated by the American Association of Colleges of Nursing (AACN). The AACN programs focus on curriculum development and creating careers in advanced practice geriatric nursing.

"We work collaboratively to coordinate the resources and information generated within each program and to develop a network of support for this building workforce in geriatric nursing. In September 2005, Dr. Claire Fagin, the BAGNC Program Director for the first five years, and I published an article in *Imprint Magazine*, the publication for the National Student Nurses Association, highlighting five scholars and fellows and why they chose geriatric nursing. We want nurses who are just beginning their professional career to recognize geriatric nursing as an exciting field with extraordinary career potential."

Patty affirms the necessity of making changes at the systems level. Toward that goal, the JAHF Board offered scholarships to nurses interested in administration and enrolled in MBA programs. These scholars are prepared to lead agencies and programs that provide services and care to the elderly population.

Agreeing with what Bill Thomas emphasizes in his book, *What Are Old People For?*, Patty affirms the positive impact elders have on the culture. "I think it is a grievous error if we do not value the wisdom and experience that elders represent. Programs of civic engagement can utilize resources of this population in meeting not only the needs in community, but their needs as well. The Atlantic Philanthropies in partnership with the Gerontological Society of America (GSA) Policy Institute funds and manages a civic engagement program" (http://www.geron.org/).

Patty notes that former Presidents George Bush and Bill Clinton's involvement in fund-raising for hurricanes Katrina and Rita are examples of active engagement by tapping into their considerable skills. Both former President Jimmy and Roselyn Carter have given years of additional service.

"However, the tragedy of hurricane Katrina shows that our systems aren't prepared to respond to vulnerable populations, including the elderly in nursing homes who were abandoned. The fiery bus accident in Texas during the evacuation prior to hurricane Rita revealed that elders were being transported inappropriately." Patty does not believe that society's systems problems are limited to the elderly. "When we look at Homeland Security, we must look at all populations and their needs, and that's not just the elderly, but anyone with special issues, such as mobility, whether they are [individuals] 20, 40 or 80 who will need transportation support. Having that perspective will help everybody."

The John A. Hartford Foundation Institute for Geriatric Nursing at New York University College of Nursing

Elaine Gould, MSW

Since 1996, The John A. Hartford Foundation Institute for Geriatric Nursing (Hartford Institute), housed at the New York University College of Nursing, has been the only nurse-led institute in the country to set a national agenda to shape the quality of health care that older Americans receive by promoting the highest level of geriatric competence in all nurses. By raising the standards of nursing care, the Hartford Institute aims to ensure that people age with optimal function, comfort, and dignity. The Hartford Institute identifies, develops, and disseminates best practices in the nursing care of older adults and focuses on infusing these practices into the education of every nursing student and the work environment of every practicing professional nurse. The Hartford Institute educates the public to expect the best nursing practice and encourages national leadership to establish best practice as the standard for geriatric nursing care (www.hartfordign.org).

Elaine Gould, MSW, Director of Programs at the Hartford Institute for Geriatric Nursing, works with the Hartford Institute's director, Mathy Mezey, EdD, RN, FAAN, and co-directors Terry Fulmer, PhD, RN, FAAN, and Elizabeth Capezuti, PhD, RN, FAAN, to carry out the work of the Hartford Institute in four areas: education, practice, research, and policy.

"It is clear," says Elaine Gould, "that older adults are the core business of health care, but that reality is not something that hospitals yet fully recognize. If you look at quality indicator data that hospitals already track—such as falls, complications from medications, extended length of stay—you will find that it is the hospital's elderly patients that are the center of these data," she reports. "[However], most hospitals have yet to make a strong, specific commitment to eldercare.

"Because nurses are central to the care delivered in hospitals, they can be vital to finding solutions for providing quality hospital care to older adults. However, in order to create solutions, all hospital nurses must know the fundamentals of geriatric care, recognize geriatric syndromes, know best practices around these issues, and assess all patients with a 'geriatric lens.' Hospitals are reluctant to 'buy in to geriatrics' because there is often no focus for geriatric care in the facility. Patients can be in all parts of the hospital on all the floors. Moreover, there is no consensus on even defining a 'geriatric patient.' Is it age, a certain level of infirmity, or comorbid conditions?"

According to Elaine, the Institute is working on several fronts to address such issues. "We have the Nurses Improving Care to Health-system Elders Program (NICHE), where hospitals make a commitment to providing high quality eldercare. There are 157 hospitals around the country to date that have committed to NICHE. There are nurse-led models of care that these hospitals initiate. Two of the most popular models are the geriatric resource nurse (GRN), where nurses become unit-based resources in geriatric best practices, and the Acute Care for the Elderly (ACE) Units, where geriatric patients receive comprehensive coordinated care often led by geriatric nurse practitioners in collaboration with geriatricians," she explains.

"The American Organization of Nurse Executives (AONE) is undertaking a new initiative with the Hartford Institute to develop the concept 'Elder-Friendly Hospitals,'" Elaine notes. "The Nurse Competence in Aging Project (NCA), which is a joint venture with the American Nurses Association (ANA) and the American Nurses Credentialing Center (ANCC) and funded by the Atlantic Philanthropies through American Nurses Foundation (ANF), targets 57 national specialty associations to enhance geriatric information within their nursing specialty. NCA created a comprehensive geriatric nursing Web site (www.geronurseonline.org) and encourages gerontological certification. Lastly, the Hartford Institute provides a variety of resource materials such as a Best Practices CD-ROM with 20 geriatric-topic modules of PowerPoint slides, a series of assessment instruments called *Try This,* and delineated geriatric competencies for hospital nurses available to staff development educators to help them introduce defined competencies and geriatric best practices [in]to their continuing education activities, performance evaluations, and JCAHO [Joint Commission on Accreditation of Healthcare Organizations] reporting."

The idea that older adults are health care's core business is not limited to work in hospitals. It is the basis for all of the Hartford Institute's work in nursing education as well, according to Elaine. "Nursing students need to enter the workforce competent to care for the patients they will encounter. A National Council of State Boards of Nursing survey found that new nurses report that the majority of their patients are over the age of 65. Yet, nursing schools are only now beginning to recognize the importance of geriatric content in their curricula. The Hartford Institute conducted two national surveys in 1996 and 2003 found that while there are substantial improvements, less than one-third of the schools had a required free-standing course in geriatrics. The main reasons they cited for lack of content were 'no room in the curriculum' or 'the lack of competent faculty to teach geriatrics.' However, these are merely excuses," she believes. "A change in priorities creates solutions and a commitment to a 'geriatric lens.' Staff development educators frequently state that they have to 'teach geriatrics' to their new nurses. This is a clear statement of the need for curricular change," she states firmly.

Elaine believes that it is important for nursing instructors to understand that there are teaching and learning moments in geriatrics, particularly if faculty are attempting to integrate material into a particular course. "For example," she recounts, "when instructors teach the use of catheters and IVs, they often mention pediatric implications. However, students also need to know about the geriatric implications of catheters and IVs. Such moments become evident when a faculty member uses a 'geriatric lens' to look at curriculum. One doesn't have to have a major curriculum redesign to incorporate this knowledge; there are many teaching moments where geriatric information can be added. Many faculty members tend to believe they must be experts when including such material, but there is a difference between being comfortable and being an authority. We believe nursing faculty need enough knowledge to be comfortable introducing such material."

Along with many others we interviewed for this book, Elaine believes that behind this historical neglect of geriatric education stands the perception that elders are of lesser value in our culture. "Fortunately, it is getting much better in nursing schools," she relates, "because The John A. Hartford Foundation has made a multimillion dollar commitment to enhance geriatric education in nursing schools, and the American Association of Colleges of Nursing (AACN) has made a major commitment to geriatric education.

"Along with AACN, The Hartford Institute has been working on several fronts to address the need to enhance geriatric content in baccalaureate nursing curriculum. Together, The Hartford Institute and AACN have created a baccalaureate geriatric competencies document to supplement AACN's Essentials Competencies. Subsequently, AACN published a geriatric competencies document for advanced practice nursing. These are all available on the AACN Web site" (www.aacn.nche.edu).

Elaine adds, "Many schools already have made a substantial commitment to incorporating geriatrics into their curriculum through free-standing required courses, substantive integrated content, innovative clinical experiences, and dedicated faculty. AACN and the Hartford Institute created a series of national awards showcasing geriatric nursing excellence at schools. These awards, presented at AACN's national deans' meeting, highlight the importance of geriatrics as an area of expertise and raise the bar of competence in the field. Summaries of the various award-winning curricula can be found on their Web sites, www.hartfordign.org and www.aacn.nche.edu.

"The award-winning curricula feature, for example, didactic courses that encourage activities so that students understand the psychological complexity of growing older. The clinical experiences often expose students to a range of healthy as well as frail elders so that students can see a broad spectrum of elder health issues. In addition, because many nursing students experience their first clinical rotation in nursing homes and hospitals where their patients are predominantly elderly, some programs have changed the introductory life span course to be taught 'backwards,' starting with geriatrics and ending with pediatrics to give the students some knowledge in the care of older adults before they enter their first clinical setting."

According to Elaine, the Hartford Institute has also developed materials that nursing programs can utilize to enhance geriatric education, providing modules that can help create full, independent courses, or when used separately, can be integrated into current curricular offerings. There is a CD-ROM, similar to the one prepared for staff development educators, entitled *Best Nursing Practices in Care For Older Adults*. There are content modules and a curriculum guide developed by geriatric nursing experts that provide faculty with ready-made text and audiovisuals. The Institute has found that the *Try This* series, noted above, has been very useful for faculty as well as staff development educators. The Hartford Institute disseminates these materials at AACN conferences and on its Web site, www.hartfordign.org.

With funding from the John A. Hartford Foundation, AACN is initiating additional and substantial faculty development to enhance upper-level baccalaureate curricula. The Hartford Institute will be creating resources for this project. The Hartford Institute also attends the AACN conference to enhance faculty expertise and disseminate resources.

"The Hartford Institute recently completed a study looking at the Web sites of AACN member schools," Elaine reports, "to see how older adults are portrayed pictorially. Not surprisingly, what we found is that there are many more pictures of nurses with babies than elders. This imagery is unfortunate, because it creates a disconnect between the patients that new students think they will care for as a nurse and the population that they will actually encounter when they graduate. Generally, when people enter nursing school, they think that the profession is about caring for babies, children, and younger adults, but that is only a small part of nursing. Roughly 50% of all hospital beds are filled by people 65 or older."

Although the Hartford Institute generally focuses primarily on hospitals and education, it has done some work in long-term care and assisted living. The Institute has created staffing level recommendations and developed recommendations for the role of advanced practice nurses in nursing homes. It is now engaged in defining elements of a high quality "teaching nursing home" and in crosswalking geriatric competencies of several professions: nurses, social workers, physicians, dentists, pharmacists, and nursing home administrators. It has also explored the role of nursing in assisted living.

Elaine has personal as well as professional experience in geriatrics and long-term care from her responsibilities of managing the care of her 93-year-old mother. Elaine believes long-term care should be based upon individual needs and allow for flexibility as needs change over time. "Socialization is also very important for quality of life. But, long-term care centers around maximizing autonomy and function. However, this is easier for professionals to accomplish than for family members. Maximizing autonomy takes time and patience. For example, nurses in home care can spend that extra time to maximize function because that is often an important part of a care plan. But for family caregivers, maximizing autonomy and function can increase risk and reduce caregiving efficiency, creating far greater emotional and time demands on the responsible family member."

She observes, "Think of a continuum when giving care, from total autonomy at one end to total dependence at the other. Obviously, most caregiving falls in between the two extremes, and this is where we struggle. For family caregiving, it becomes a struggle between an elder's desire for autonomy and a family member's need for efficiency. Emotions of both the elder and their children often complicate the process, an issue not as significant for the professional caregiver. To complicate matters even more, as people are living longer, there is an increased prevalence of what I call 'double or even triple geriatric families,' where the mother is 95, the daughter is 77 and the granddaughter is 55."

Elaine suggests several outstanding literature sources on long-term care and family caregiving. "Ethel Mitty, EdD, RN, based at the NYU College of Nursing, is one of the leaders in nursing care management in nursing homes and in understanding a nurse's role in assisted living environments. Carol Levine, Director of Families and Health Care Project, United Hospital Fund of New York, has written extensively on the trials and tribulations of family caregiving and the excruciating consequences of health care policy on family caregiving."

Elaine Gould's specific geriatric interest is in healthcare professionals' abilities to communicate effectively with older adults. "There are physical, cognitive, psychological, and social barriers that interfere with effective communication. Caregivers must recognize the differences between normal aging and pathological issues and recognize that sensory loss in older adults is a huge problem. Some people can't hear, see, chew, or move well. These conditions are not necessarily life threatening, but they have enormous impact on quality of life and on communicating with elders whether in assessment, treatment, or teaching settings. All these sensory losses lead to frustration, which in turn leads to either aggressive or withdrawing behaviors, making communication difficult," explains Elaine. "Moreover, even though someone may be cognitively intact, cognitive learning slows down, making multitasking difficult. Older adults also have psychological and social baggage that often interferes with their ability to communicate. It is the healthcare professional's responsibility to foster optimal function and find common ground in the communication interaction."

On the leading edge of aging baby boomers herself, Elaine Gould joins an increasing number of pioneers working to enhance eldercare and to expand grassroots clinical geriatric knowledge.

BEACON OF CARE

Sarah H. Kagan, PhD, RN

"What is old?" asks Sarah H. Kagan, Associate Professor and Doris R. Schwartz Term Professor in Gerontological Nursing at the University of Pennsylvania School of Nursing. "Except for those who may suffer from a chronic condition or disease, the general perception is that someone in their sixties or early seventies is really not old," she states. "Many people can't give a particularly apt definition of what is old, which I believe represents a kind of crossroads in our society. Toward that end, I am very optimistic that we are in a time of flux where people are reevaluating their perceptions about aging."

Sarah believes that the climate surrounding aging is shifting in a positive manner, in part because of the changing demographics. "It's difficult to maintain a climate of overt discrimination and 'elder bashing' when so many people know and love someone who is considered an older adult by [the] usual criterion of an age of about 65. We are seeing more publications, media campaigns, and advertising aimed at people over the age of 55, and most especially people over 65 and 75 years old. Just now in Philadelphia we have a new aging campaign produced by our Area Agency on Aging directed toward protecting older adults and their families from elder scams, which have become major problems in recent years."

Sarah's interest in the field of gerontology and eldercare grew out of finishing a bachelor's degree in behavioral science. "Between my third and fourth years in college, I worked on the farm where I grew up as a child," she relates. "I was reflecting upon my career options and knew that I liked older folks. After spending one summer caring for an older friend of the family, I realized that gerontological nursing made sense and was socially significant.

"I'm lucky to be doing what I love—caring for older adults and their families—and learning from them so that I can share this knowledge and develop or investigate better ways of caring. My special interests in the care of older adults who have cancer allow me the intimate privilege of being with patients at the best and worst times of their lives. That intimacy acts as a beacon—it reminds me of the value that

I, and nursing as a profession, contribute to society, and [of] the rewards offered in return," she maintains.

Sarah firmly believes that, as a society, we still have significant challenges ahead in meeting the needs of an aging population. On a sociopolitical level, we have a difficult time understanding the magnitude of health and social care needs. Chronic illness is rapidly emerging as a concern, including the individual and social disabilities attached to such infirmities. They weigh heavily upon our society in a variety of socioeconomic, personal, and familial ways. "Just think about someone with Alzheimer's disease and all of the care involved on the part of family, friends, professional caregivers, and institutions like assisted living facilities or the family's place of worship," she says.

Sarah underscores that many issues attach themselves to such challenges, such as limited health and social services, of which many available today seem poorly integrated one with another. In addition, limited training opportunities exist for clinicians as well as for health and social service workers who are not professionals but who assist older adults. And, of course, a paramount issue for this latter group involves concerns around adequate compensation and other matters of quality work life. Although they represent the backbone of services, personal care workers find themselves dramatically underpaid.

"I personally prefer to view such issues in terms of options and opportunities as opposed to problems," Sarah emphasizes. "I tend to take to task our policy makers, administrators, and educators because we have known about the demographics for a long period of time. Perceptions haven't changed but have simply grown in magnitude before our very eyes. For example, in medicine and nursing, we've been talking about preparing student clinicians to provide health care for an aging population. However, until recently, for the most part, the focus centered on training specialists in geriatric nursing and medicine whose domain is largely the realm of caring for so-called 'frail elders.' But, promoting specialists and specialization implies that we are dealing with a relatively rare or minor problem, not something common across the board. One of the things we know about health care is that most of the people who use healthcare services are chronologically, biologically or functionally older. It makes little sense to train specialists alone when the issues of the aging population impact us all," she states emphatically.

For this reason, Sarah champions the position that every physician, nurse, and all other healthcare providers, including physical therapists and speech and language pathologists, need foundational exposure to aging content and knowledge of care for older adults. She states that gerontological courses have been a part of only some nursing curricula. At a national level, educational policy statements from the John A. Hartford Institute for Geriatric Nursing and the American Association of Colleges of Nursing have emphasized required undergraduate courses in all curricula for close to a decade; this is not a new specialty, yet curricula have not consistently reflected that fact.

"Today we have a foundational understanding of what it means to age, and it needs to be shared with almost all caregivers," Sarah believes. "Even in pediatrics, one can run into aging issues. Someone may have a grandmother caring for grandchildren because their mother is ill or working. Regardless of age or socioeconomic conditions, almost any family is likely to experience a time, even for a short period, when they are caring for a person of advanced age."

Sarah is convinced that professional education for healthcare providers must be more specific than broad-brushed. For example, psychological and social sciences reveal many aspects of the aging process and underscore that it is diverse and complicated at multiple levels. Physiological aging is equally complex and far less explored. For example, what we perceive to be the appearance of looking old is mediated by environmental factors such as exposure to radiation from the sun. This environmental exposure is likely more consequential than intrinsic aging changes in the skin itself. For other organ systems, however, the balance between environmental effects and innate changes over time may be very different. That balance is difficult to investigate and document as life patterns and exposures vary widely from individual to individual.

Sarah believes that it is critical for caregivers to examine their own preconceptions of what it means to be old, many of which are incorrect. She remarks, "We continue to grapple with well-intended parental notions about appropriate interactions with older adults. With all the best intentions, many people enjoy working with older adults but often refer to them as a parent addresses a child, engaging in behaviors that belie an older person's maturity and wisdom. Though well-intentioned, people frequently use words like 'dear' or 'sweetie' and may go beyond patronizing speech in attempting to speak for the older person. Such language is often used without knowing the particular background or personality of the individual. Inappropriate preconceptions can also be corrected through foundational education about the aging process."

In addition, for a very long period, healthcare providers, especially nurses, have presumed that gerontological nursing centers upon the care of frail institutionalized older adults. "It's been thought that the easiest way to teach basic nursing fundamentals is with such individuals," Sarah postulates. "I think this is inappropriate! In reality, the care of older, frail adults in nursing homes is one of the most complicated healthcare specialties. It is intensely intellectually demanding and requires a high level of skill, because we are dealing with a group of people for whom diseases and other problems are likely to be complex and insidious. Because of their longevity, social and psychological needs are likely to be equally involved. Plus, we must keep in mind that only about 5% of older adults live in such facilities at any given time.

"I would like to see the day in entry-level nursing education where we don't expose first-year students to the care of older adults in residential facilities. I envision a time when placement in a long-term care facility is offered to nursing students who have met significant standards of preparation. Caring for the aging and the aged becomes the goal, an achievement, and not a default entry position."

Sarah proposes that we need a new, social dialogue about what it means to be old and to face the prospect of our own mortality. "Our society seems to be stuck in a kind of adolescent belief that life goes on forever. It's much easier to talk about sex than it is to speak about death!"

PASSIONATE NURSE EDUCATOR

Anne Vanderbilt, RN, MSN

When asked why she remains in the often-chaotic healthcare arena, Anne Vanderbilt responds, "I still really love the nursing profession as a whole. I believe that nursing serves as the best way to impact patients in a caring and positive manner. This perception is supported by national surveys indicating that nursing is one of the most trusted careers."

As a clinical nurse specialist in geriatric nursing at the Cleveland Clinic Foundation in Cleveland, Ohio, her primary role is that of instructor, teaching other nurses about the discipline. She informs us that older people, much like children, have specialty conditions that affect them more commonly than others. Unlike the field of pediatrics, unfortunately only a small percentage of nurses are trained in geriatrics, although the numbers are rising.

Geriatric nursing differs from the typical nursing model, believes Anne. "The focus is different. Elders have more special needs, and the way they present as patients is different. Understanding these differences is important in how we care for them. We have to be sensitive to how they are affected by medications. We must be careful to examine our goals. Often when elders enter the hospital, the essential focus is not upon finding a cure. Rather, caring may mean offering a person more comfort and increased ability to function, and their issues may revolve around increasing quality of life. Discharge planning that takes into account their family dynamics is important. Unfortunately, this may result in some healthcare professionals experiencing diminished satisfaction in terms of the traditional medical model."

Anne participates in a program called Nurses Improving Care for Health System Elders (NICHE) (www.hartfordign.org/programs/niche), mentioned earlier. The just over 150 hospitals participating in the program report the following outcomes:

- Enhanced nursing knowledge and skills regarding treatment of common geriatric syndromes;
- Greater patient satisfaction;

- Decreased length of stay for elderly patients;
- Reductions in readmission rates;
- Increases in the length of time between readmissions; and
- Reductions in costs associated with hospital care for the elderly

Anne became a nurse because of the influence of her mother, who is also a nurse. "She remained home with me during my earlier years, and then returned to the profession when I entered junior high school," explains Anne. "She enjoyed her work and had many funny stories to tell. I also liked the sciences during school and especially biology. After graduating from nursing school and taking the traditional path of working in a hospital, I eventually entered a period of self-assessment determining what I liked and did not like about the profession. That is when I decided to return to school and to focus upon elders. I especially enjoyed the teaching aspect of nursing, teaching patients and families as well as peers."

Prior to her employment at the Cleveland Clinic, Anne worked in a long-term care facility as a nurse practitioner and as a staff development coordinator. She brings this experience to her current job and appreciates the clinic's general trend toward more holistic health care, including the use of such modalities as guided imagery and relaxation techniques. In addition, nationwide, hospital units serving the elderly are being structurally changed. For example, some units have been modified to make communal dining possible, also having rooms that allow for more activities and space for family gatherings. Changing the physical environment gives patients more choices and greater independence.

According to Anne, we can learn from elders. "Elders teach us about patience, and their many life experiences give them a unique perspective. Older people, especially when they are sick and in the hospital, do things much more slowly. We have a tendency to want to hurry about and speed things up, but you can't do this with elders. They tend to speak slower and move slower. They teach us the tremendous value of slowing down and not rushing. They also teach us not to take things for granted and show us the value of diversity."

Anne recalls as a new nurse caring for one patient who was 100, fairly unusual for a man. "He was highly functional and had just experienced a stroke. His 80-year-old daughter who was living with him brought him to the hospital. He came to us severely impaired, but over the first 24 hours he responded remarkably well, regaining many of his functions. He had a large family, and they were elated when he began to move again. He left the hospital, entered rehabilitation, and I lost track of him. However, within in few months he suffered another stroke and came back to the same floor as before. This time the stroke was much more devastating. He could not speak at all, which was quite disconcerting because he was an independent, feisty old man.

"The question arose about whether to use a feeding tube. Although he never signed any advanced directives, he [had] made it quite clear earlier that he did not want a feeding tube. In addition, he began to pull out the intravenous tubes. I remember sitting with him, holding his hand and sensing that he was attempting to tell us that he didn't want to live. He died a few days later. It was a very moving experience for me, and I will always remember him.

"There is a certain influential energy in having a one-on-one interaction and in the ability to make a lasting impact on patients," states Anne. "Even though today I serve in a different, educational capacity, I still periodically take on assignments and care for patients. However, my role is to assist the nurses in conducting their work. Especially with new nurses, it is very rewarding to see their growth."

Good Samaritan Society

Gail Blocker, LNHA

The Evangelical Lutheran Good Samaritan Society (Society) began in the 1920s when the Lutheran Church partnered with church leaders in small, rural communities to provide care for people who had no other options for care. Today, the society, with its national campus located in Sioux Falls, South Dakota, is the nation's largest not-for-profit long-term care organization owning or managing Christian communities of care in 24 states, employing more than 22,000 staff members and serving more than 28,000 residents. The vast majority of those served are elderly, but the Society also assists others of various ages in need. They offer housing options that include nursing beds, assisted living, basic and residential care, and senior living (individual homes, apartment units, HUD units, duplexes, and mobile homes). Healthcare services include skilled nursing, subacute and board care, and home health care along with outpatient physical, occupational, speech, respiratory, and intravenous therapies. Other special services include adult day care, specialty care units, respite care, hospice care, and home health services. Child day care along with after-school programs are also a service in several Society locations. All Society centers and services are first and foremost organized to provide a Christian ministry to residents, families, and the surrounding communities.

According to Gail Blocker, Director, Administrative Services and Education, the Society is dedicated toward an aging-in-place concept. Although senior living options are designed for elders who remain well and who are at least somewhat independent, there are resources available as frailty increases, to allow elders to remain at home as long as possible, Gail relates. "When direct care is not available, people can contract for home care resources or discuss options to keep a person safe and in their home with what is often called 'negotiated risk.' For example, it may become necessary to disengage a stove or arrange for food service, overnight live-in care, etc. This allows the risk of safety to be shared by both management and the resident or family and could keep a person in place longer."

Admittedly, the considerable financial pressures and regulatory constraints that organizations experience put pressure on the feasibility of this approach. "We have a staff person who works closely with our nation's House and Senate leaders," Gail asserts. "We also assist facility managers and administrators to become grassroot lobbyists on the state level. We encourage others in telling our story with letter writing or direct invitations to our centers to observe firsthand the quality that is provided with limited resources. We want people to understand that we provide good value for the dollar. Unfortunately, in Minnesota some of the staff have not received raises for more than three years. Yet, they continue to conscientiously do the work. Nebraska took a cut in Medicaid, so our people had to be creative and resourceful in doing things differently. In some areas, facilities exist in close proximity to one another, making it possible to do job sharing. For example, an environmental supervisor may serve more than one operation. In addition, we are looking for new technology to improve productivity and quality."

The Society held an innovation summit in 2005, looking for ways to enhance creativity and productivity. At all levels, management encourages and targets forward thinking. "Some of the nursing facilities have had to downsize, some by more than 20% and at some locations by more than 50%. We may see increased home health services or look at more assisted living, both of which do not require as many staff. This also allows people choices in where and how they receive the needed care."

One strategy to limit the silo effect (i.e., a lack of communication and common goals between departments) of services and cut down on some of the costs is to develop the "universal worker," notes Gail. As Certified Nursing Assistants (CNAs), these persons perform multiple tasks as a team, perhaps doing laundry and serving meals as well as providing personal care.

Gail now coordinates the Administrator in Training (AIT) Program for between 20 to 24 interns each year. Prior to this role she served as an Administrator for the Society for approximately 15 years in three care centers. Participants in the AIT Program rotate through each functional area of a nursing home along with other services provided at one of the Society's 240 locations. They also attend workshops on finance, human resources, quality, and spiritual leadership, as well as engage in self-paced, distance learning available through a satellite system that is available at each location. "In addition, if we have an administrator who is struggling to perform well in a particular area, I can structure personalized training and other resources for him or her," she says. Administrators can also request training suited to their specific needs, and she will try to find the resources available to them.

The Society offers a large variety of academic courses for nurses, nursing assistants, and the like. "Often, such opportunities are unavailable, especially in rural areas, so we like to call it 'growing our own,'" Gail reports.

Gail also supports organizational enhancement efforts as the Society seeks to become more innovative in its senior care. They are expanding home health care services and increasing senior living options based upon a neighborhood concept. "One of my roles involves making sure that new executive managers (executive level housing managers) support these initiatives," she underscores. "Currently, I enjoy working on developing a curriculum for senior housing. We will soon be offering a senior housing management certification program.

"People want choices," Gail believes, referring to the current aging and eldercare climate in the United States. "Residents and families alike tell us that they want us to give them alternatives. For example, they don't always want the traditional nursing home model that has existed for many years." Interestingly, she does not necessarily think that cost is the limiting factor. If they have the funds, some older adults are willing to pay more for the freedom to choose and be in their own homes or go to a more social model of care, assisted living, apartment with services, or home health services. Developing more HUD (Housing and Urban Development) housing makes it possible to offer affordable housing alternatives as HUD removes some of its previous restrictions for allowing some care services to be permitted, as many of the low-income elders apply for such housing assistance.

Although the term "strengths-based assessment" is not used per se, Gail reports that the approach is used as much as possible when new elders enter the system. "We pride ourselves on being a learning organization; we even have a 'senior college' that originates from South West Minnesota State University, Marshall, Minnesota, which is on our satellite system and then downloaded to several of our facilities, where residents can participate at scheduled times and even invite people from the community to attend sessions. The topics are almost endless and include politics, history, literature, poetry, and even building a personal history scrapbook, all based upon interests and needs assessments. Some subject-matter experts have even come to our in-house production studio to broadcast the senior college."

Spiritual care is another obvious emphasis for the Society. They begin meetings with prayer, offer Bible studies, and conduct bedside memorial services when someone dies. In terms of the latter, before a person's body is removed, family and staff are invited to attend a service as a way of sharing grief and good-byes. Gail says, "Many family members would tell me, 'This is when I said goodbye to Mother or Dad—the funeral was for everyone else.' Of course, we honor a variety of belief systems, and our centers strive at how we can best meet the needs of families and staff during this time of death and dying."

New staff members are given training in the aging process, according to Gail. "We review the aging process during our general employee orientation sessions, and in addition, we counsel staff to view each person, no matter how frail, as having a spirit and soul. Sometimes I would tell a family that they might not realize what a gift a resident has been to us, especially in terms of their wisdom and sense of humor. No offense, but because they cherish their independence and may have fewer social skills than women, men often become the most distraught when they first arrive in an extended care environment. However, many of them soon blossom and enjoy kidding and joking." She shares the story of the gentleman who wanted his glass of whiskey, which had been approved by his doctor to have each night. However, he thought it was disappearing too fast and insisted the staff was drinking it. So, every night he drew a line on the bottle and wanted me to buy his whiskey when his supply would become low. It became a kind of community joke as I went to the grocery store with a list of beverages wanted by the residents," she laughs. "In any case, it becomes a matter of building trust, then watching people begin to enjoy themselves."

Some of the Society's facilities actively pursue story gathering as a way of leaving a legacy. Partnering with schools, students assist in capturing residents' stories with tape recorders and then transcribing them. They also participate in a "Make a Wish"-type program where elders are granted the opportunity of doing something they have wanted to do, including everything from taking a hot air balloon ride to eating in a particular restaurant. One woman wanted to ride a motorcycle, so the staff contacted a local Harley-Davidson dealer to make it possible.

Retaining and motivating employees who are at the lower pay scales is financially challenging, Gail agrees. "Our turnover rate remains far below the national average," she reports proudly. "We make certain that our supervisors receive superior training, assisting employees to feel a sense of worth and purpose in their jobs. In addition, our President/CEO hosts a CNA conference each year. A select group attends, representing all 12 regions. We also have CNA-of-the-Year awards at each location. Many of our employees have extended years of service. They feel compassionate about our organization's mission.

"Of course, the work tends to be quite physically challenging. The Society allows older workers to become more specialized, doing tasks that don't require heavy lifting. We also are encouraging our centers to become no-lift centers."

In support of the Society's mission and commitment to innovation, the home care component of their service is expanding, including into more rural areas. Utilizing the federal government's program, The Programs of All-inclusive Care for the Elderly (PACE), allows them to tap into other community resources. PACE is a new benefit that features a comprehensive service delivery system and integrated Medicare and Medicaid financing combining medical, social, and long-term care services for frail people. For most participants, the comprehensive service package permits them to continue living at home while receiving services rather than be institutionalized. PACE is available only in states that have chosen to offer it under Medicaid. "A client turns over Medicare and Medicaid resources to a case manager, who makes sure that personal needs are met. Again, people want choices, and PACE becomes a means to provide them."

Case managers may also find it helpful to utilize the Internet's BenefitsCheckUp program sponsored by the National Council on Aging (www.benefitscheckup.com). BenefitsCheckUp is the nation's most comprehensive online service to screen for federal, state, and some local private and public benefits for older adults (ages 55 and over). It contains over 1,300 different programs from all 50 states (including the District of Columbia). On average there are 50 to 70 programs available to individuals per state. Every day, it helps thousands of people connect to government programs that can help them pay for prescription drugs, health care, utilities, and other needs.

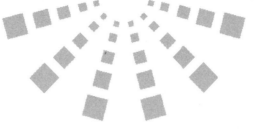

Section 5
Spirituality and Aging

"Young men's minds are always changeable, but when an old man is concerned in a matter, he looks both before and after"

—Homer, *The Iliad*

*I*n This Section . . . Wise care providers understand that many elders embrace a sense of cosmic communion. Through numerous faith traditions, elders may experience a time of deepening spiritual awareness and growth.

SACRED AT ANY AGE

Rabbi Cary Kozberg

"Every life is sacred," states Rabbi Cary Kozberg emphatically, a basic message that he wants to communicate to all eldercare providers. Cary is currently the Director of Religious Life Council for Jewish Elderly in Chicago. Formerly he was the chaplain at the Wexner Heritage Village in Columbus, Ohio, a Jewish not-for-profit provider of health, housing, social, and spiritual services primarily serving older adults and persons with disabilities. He reports that the issues facing the elders who live at the village are real and genuine. "These people are living at a time in their lives when politics don't matter much anymore, nor do they display what Ecclesiastes calls 'vanity.' Along with their families, they often struggle to keep things together every day."

Throughout his career, Cary has been drawn to ministering to people who have been marginalized in one form or another or who are facing a period of transition, a pattern that certainly holds true as he serves frail older adults and individuals suffering from dementia. "Unfortunately, our society writes these people off as having little or no value," he reports sadly. "My prophetic stance underscores that, in essence, these are people like the rest of us. Because I am one of them, it will be interesting to see how the baby boomers deal with old age issues. I don't believe they will put up with the current environment."

Within the context of the Jewish faith tradition and in light of frailty and other forms of human suffering, he believes that we need to recover sacred anger. "We are often told that we must accept whatever comes our way," he observes. "Of course, there is a time for such acceptance, but there is also a time to challenge hardships and to express one's vitality through frustration and anger. In scripture, Job serves as a penetrating example, a faithful and righteous man who nonetheless suffered greatly. There is also a Hasidic tradition of challenging God based upon the idea that, if we are in covenant partnership with God, the relationship becomes intimate enough for us to express many thoughts and forms of emotion. The definition of Israel is 'one who wrestles with God,' a very powerful image."

Cary's comments remind us of a story about Mother Teresa. One day as she was crossing a river on a cart, something broke down and she found herself waist deep in water. She wagged her finger at the sky, saying, "If this is how you treat your friends, no wonder you have so few of them."

Traditionally in Judaism, elders enjoyed an honored position. Today, however, Cary perceives such revered status as more of an ideal. He states, "In Leviticus we are called to honor the elderly. My sense is that if we honored the elderly in a natural way, the commandment would be unnecessary. Because God commands it, honoring elders is not something we do naturally. In any case, when we affirm elderhood, we find ourselves being affirmed.

"Interestingly, there is also a verse in scripture juxtaposed to Leviticus speaking about treating the stranger in our midst. In our society, older adults frequently find themselves being treated as strangers. They are not respected and accepted unless they have a lot of money or power. Marginalized, society makes fun of them."

The frequent supposedly humorous elder-focused e-mails making the rounds perpetuate this attitude, such as:

"I'm a walking storeroom of facts but I've just lost the key to the storeroom door."

"You know you are old when you order stewed prunes and your waiter says, 'Excellent choice!'"

Reflecting on his broad view of spirituality, Cary explains his perspective. "First, for me, holiness is found in relationships such as the ones described by Jewish theologian Martin Buber in his book, 'I and Thou.' Buber focuses on the way humans relate to their world. By simply observing, measuring, and examining people and things, we keep ourselves detached from meaningful relationships in an 'I-it' stance. On the other hand, it is possible to place ourselves completely into a relationship, to truly understand and to be present with another person, which he describes in terms of 'I-Thou'" (Buber 1923, p. 4).

Continuing, Cary asserts, "Secondly, holy connections are found in the spaces 'in between.' I have a picture of Michelangelo's creation where God is stretching out His hand. However, the picture offers no image of God or man, but contains only the two arms with the center being the space in between. Another image that comes to mind is the space between the two cherubim on the Ark of the Covenant. For me, we experience God in these spaces, which represent times of transition. For example, the symbolic 'space in between' leaving one's home and entering a long-term care facility can be very traumatic. To ease the transition, we have a welcoming service every month or so for new long-term residents and their families. We believe that moving into a long-term care residence is a life cycle passage. We put together a service of readings, poetry, etc. which acknowledges the sorrow and the anxiety, but also expresses hope."

During such times of transition, we might wish to keep in mind the Chinese understanding of the word *crisis*, which means both *danger* and *opportunity*. Rituals like the one Cary mentions may help us to view a transition as a call to a new experience as well as a loss. "By faith Abraham obeyed when he was called to a [new] place" (Hebrews 11:8 RSV). Like Abraham, there are new freedoms to be found in leaving home, in many instances freedom from the isolation of living alone and the freedom to become friends with new people. There is the freedom of *being* as opposed to the many household *doing* chores. Although not usually perceived this way in our culture, becoming more dependent upon others also brings with it the freedom of receiving needed gifts and services.

We also recommend that family and friends join in a "good-bye" ritual, videotaping an elder's home or at least taking pictures, as well as joining in other activities such as reminiscing. Just as there are rituals for the blessing of a new home, perhaps clergy and others in one's support community could be enlisted to engage in a ceremony of good grief and thanksgiving.

"Of course, birth and death often become the most powerful transitions," Cary reminds us. "When a resident dies or is in the dying process at Wexner, our Jewish perspective guides our end-of-life rituals. Memorial services are conducted for both family and staff. If a staff member is particularly close to a resident and her/his family, we encourage them to attend the funeral and [at the service] to share the[ir] experiences they had with the deceased."

The question of what happens to people after death varies among faith traditions. Robert J. Kastenbaum describes several long-standing and newly emerging interpretations in *Death, Society, and Human Experience:*

- Death is an enfeebled form of life. In this scenario, people are tired, sad, bored, suffering, and don't have much to do, perhaps depicted by Morley in *Scrooge.*
- Death is a continuation of more of the same. A number of tribal societies view this as a recycling process.
- The universe is a realm of perpetual development, so we continue to evolve in one form or another in one of many universes in the overall cosmos. The body may die, but consciousness lives on.
- There is nothing after death. Each person has only one life to live; what you see is what you get.
- Death is a sleep-like state from which we awaken at the final Day of Judgment (Kastenbaum 2004).

According to Cary, there are basically two Jewish viewpoints about life after death. "Many Jewish people are either ambivalent about it or don't believe in an afterlife. The history behind this disconnect may have to do with how Jews have reacted to living in a sometimes very harsh, aggressive Christian environment. However, the truth behind the Christian concept of reward and punishment after this life comes from a strongly held Rabbinic idea. Traditional Jewish theology definitely teaches that there is life after death. Our prayer book affirms that this life is not ended at death, that God doesn't abandon us at the end. This stance enhances a sense of hope in people and heightens their ability to cope with everyday challenges."

Cary finds in his experience that not all healthcare providers are cognizant of elderhood processes and issues. The training of nurses and, to some extent, of social workers, appears to be essentially clinical and task-oriented in nature. Although some people have a natural talent for getting the entire picture of caring for elders, he observes that caregivers seem to be limited in their service orientation. "For this reason, along with the Director of Social Services and our continuing education coordinator, we are planning to design programs that promote a more holistic vision and practice," Cary underscores. "We hope people will become internally motivated to engage in sacred work. We want them to not only focus upon how to do their work, but why they do it in the sense of having a mission and calling. Eldercare is not like flipping burgers are Wendy's," he says emphatically.

Eldercare providers at many levels communicate the belief in the sacredness of life, he notes. "The worse thing you can do is to call someone a vegetable," he says, referring to the 2005 Terry Schiavo case that received national media attention. "Although not old, Terry lay unresponsive in a Florida nursing facility for a number of years while her husband and her parents fought over her future. Regardless of one's position about her living or dying, it bothered me terribly to hear people using the terms 'persistent vegetative state.' The phrase steals away a person's humanity and leads to indifferent behavior. It says a lot about our culture, suggesting that people's lives have relative value. Rather, their lives have absolute, unconditional worth. In addition, individuals with dementia and those like Terry have much to teach us."

MINISTRY OF POSITIVE PRESENCE

Kenneth L. Nolen, MDiv

A hospital administrator once told Chaplain Ken Nolen that things are just calmer when he is on the floor. "I call that a ministry of positive presence—when you carry God's presence with you. A good friend of mine is a Catholic Priest, and he embodies God's presence. People gain assurance from that sense of presence."

Ken's perception squares with that of a growing body of people who view spirituality (and health care) more holistically, that we ultimately cannot separate the sacred from the secular. Popular author and educator Parker Palmer in his book, *Let Your Life Speak,* says it well when he describes the way to God as being "down" (Palmer 1999, p. 69). "I always imagined God to be in the same general direction as everything else I valued: up [as in upbeat or uptown]. I had failed to appreciate the meaning of some words that had intrigued me since I first heard them in seminary—[twentieth-century theologian Paul] Tillich's description of God as the 'ground of being.' I had to be forced underground before I could understand that the way to God is not up but down. Or, to put it in the words of another honored mystic, Meister Eckhart, 'God is at home [present]. It is we who have gone for a walk.'"

Twenty years in the military would not appear to lead to a second career as a chaplain. "But," explains Ken," it's one of those God things—God's plan. Life seems to be full of them. I'm not sure exactly why I decided on the chaplaincy," he says. "I knew that when I retired from the military I wanted to begin another career where I could help people. I remember once when I was lying in a hospital bed that the man in the bed next to me received a visit from a military chaplain. I recall thinking how nice it would have been to have had a visit from a chaplain myself, so I began exploring the idea of becoming one." Encouraged by one of his mentors, he began chaplaincy training after leaving the service.

Although Ken's roots are in the Episcopal Church, his ordination as a chaplain came through the International Church of the Foursquare Gospel (which is an interdenominational denomination). At the time he was completing his training, there were more chaplains looking for positions than there were openings. Advised by one of his mentors that there was always an opening for an outstanding chaplain, he determined to be the best. And, although his goal had not been to work in health care, that is where a job opened up. "Another one of those God plans," he says smiling.

Like Ken, many testimonies from people within religious traditions as well as those from other viewpoints support the notion that God has a plan for us. James Hillman, a Jungian psychologist and prolific author, states, "There is more to life than our theories of it allow. Sooner or later something seems to call us onto a particular path" (Hillman 1996, p. 3). In his book, *Callings: Finding and Following an Authentic Life*, Greg Levoy discusses methods to invoke calling into one's life, using art, pilgrimage, myth, and memory to help it to emerge into consciousness. He proclaims, "The purpose of calls is to summon adherents away from their daily grinds to a new level of awareness, into a sacred frame of mind, into communion with that which is bigger than themselves" (Levoy 1997, p. 2).

Today, Ken splits his time as a Spiritual Care Supervisor for Lucerne Hospital, one of the hospitals within the Orlando Regional Healthcare system, and is the Spiritual Care Department Educator, responsible for planning educational programs for hospital staff and the community. "We offer a number of educational programs for community clergy and spiritual caregivers, as well as continuing education for chaplains and other members of our hospital system. Just recently we held an ethics symposium for the community and were able to offer continuing education credit for nurses. Most of our programs also provide information to the attendees on preparation for impending illness and death. As a society, I don't think we do a good job of planning for such eventualities. So, we offer information and encourage people to begin thinking about having healthcare surrogates and Do Not Resuscitate orders. When people are more informed and prepared, they experience a sense of relief to know that things are taken care of. At the time of death, this preparedness enables the family to make arrangements easier and to focus on their grief and bereavement."

Lucerne has a large rehabilitation unit and typically serves an older population. In his pastoral care role, Ken usually makes rounds to patients, or he may be referred by a staff member to visit a specific patient. "I'm there to check out their spiritual concerns from an interfaith perspective," he says. "There are distinct differences between a chaplain and a community clergy person," he explains. "A chaplain must be inclusive, relating to people where they are without impinging on their particular religious backgrounds. So, we deal with people of all different faiths, from Catholic, to Jewish, to Moslem, to others. If people have their own clergy person, then that individual can be called to visit. But, more and more denominations have fewer people who can spend time visiting, and patients' hospital stays are getting shorter," he notes.

Ken's remarks remind us of a metaphor for inclusivity. Groups of people of various religious persuasions are camped at different places around the base of a huge mountain, tasked with the challenge of climbing to the top, symbolizing enlightenment. As they progress on their journeys, they begin to come closer to one another, within shouting distance, and sometimes (perhaps often) they argue about whose path to the top is better than the others. However, as they approach the top of the mountain, maturing and broadening their viewpoints as they emerge above the tree line, they become more inclusive until, upon reaching the top and seeing a more panoramic (and holistic) view, their differences virtually vanish.

Ken also supervises lay volunteers at Lucerne Hospital who feel called to work in a healthcare setting. "Volunteers receive Stephen Ministry training and also attend an Orlando Regional Healthcare spiritual care volunteer training program. They assist the chaplain, but do not administer sacraments nor do they perform assessments. Their role is to connect with families and patients, after which they may then ask a chaplain to visit."

As a society, Ken believes that we are less churched, but still are religious, partly because of the influx from other countries and different cultures. Chaplains are trained to deal with spirituality as a whole, which he describes as being engrained in every human. "We need that connection to make life worth living," he affirms. "We have a relationship with humans and a relationship with God. Both have to be fulfilled.

"I think that people over the age of 65 are somewhat more spiritual due to their own feeling of mortality," Ken suggests. "As they age, they often begin a life review, thinking about their spiritual connections, what they have missed with their family and friends, and whether they have a connection with God. They are especially concerned about establishing care for their families. As a chaplain, I listen and encourage people to talk. I use different words, based on their age differences, that may not be specifically religious."

Ken describes his job as embodying mystery. He recounts the story of a fortyish-year-old woman who had been diagnosed with very serious cancer and was scheduled for exploratory surgery the next day. "I was requested to visit with her, and she asked to have prayer. I prayed what I thought to be a normal prayer. When I went back the following day I learned that when they took her to x-ray before surgery, no cancer was found. Was that a miracle? Who knows, but I felt privileged to have participated in whatever happened."

Psychiatrist and Episcopal priest Dr. Ruth Barnhouse addressed the issue of prayer and miracles in one of her courses at Southern Methodist University's Perkins School of Theology. Two students in the class reported having relatives who were seriously ill. The class prayed for both of them. One relative quickly recovered from his illness and the other subsequently died, spurring the obvious question of whether one set of prayers was answered and the other petitions denied. Prayer, Dr. Barnhouse maintained, is not pulling some divine string in order to get God's attention. We have at best a foggy notion of how prayers are answered, let alone what happens to us after death. In the totality of God's purpose, we might assume that both prayers were answered, but not necessarily in accordance with our desire for continued life on earth.

Over the years, many elders have shared their stories with Ken. "I've met World War II fighter pilots and even a general of NORAD [North American Aerospace Defense Command]. Often people don't take the time to listen to elders; they may be busy caring for the diagnosis. But, when we listen to their stories, we gain a sense of our own mortality."

Ken has found many instances of humor in his work. He laughs when recalling a story early in his career. "I had just begun working as a chaplain and was visiting a woman in her eighties when a physician resident came in and told her he needed to check her heart. Well, right then, she simply raised her gown. What she said was, 'You've taken away my clothes and privacy; don't take away my dignity, please.'"

As a caregiver, Ken knows the importance of caring for himself and maintaining a sense of community by staying connected with fellow chaplains and within his own church. "I have a good connection with my immediate family, and I am an avid reader," he says. "If I were to offer people advice on how to age well, it would be this: First live your life to the fullest and second, while living, make relationships."

ELDER SPIRITUALITY AND CARE FOR THE COGNITIVELY IMPAIRED

Marty Richards, MSW

Marty Richards' service to elders spans more than 40 years serving as a volunteer, family member, social worker, and consultant. As a college student, she was expected to give back to the local community, so she spent four years conducting worship services in nursing homes. As a result of this experience and her ongoing work, she gained considerable knowledge about spirituality in older adults and learned how to conduct "adaptive" worship services for people with dementia. As opposed to the more traditional pattern of hymns, scripture reading, and a 20-minute sermon, she offers what some might call a "hymn sandwich," involving a hymn, scripture reading, and prayer repeated several times. She selects hymns which are well known to the particular audience, especially using ones that were popular during their youth. In addition, she encourages the use of a variety of familiar symbols such as crosses, clerical collars, and prayer shawls that communicate being connected to a community of faith.

Marty confirms the perception of many of the interviewees for this book that while an elder experiences physical and cognitive decline, their spiritual and emotional functions may remain intact. "The spiritual dimension must be accessed through the emotions as opposed to placing so much emphasis upon 'the word,'" she exclaims. "The word does not get through to a cognitively impaired person as much as music, the taste of a communion wafer, or human touch. Some clergy in more liturgical traditions become reluctant to offer communion to those who do not understand it, but my reply is, 'Who does understand it?' Different levels of understanding apart from mental processes exist, and elders are perhaps more often able to embrace the mystery behind communion."

Marty claims that often it is quite difficult for people of faith to practice rituals in a nursing home environment, especially when sharing a small room with another elder and because activities are often structured around the needs of the staff. Yet because of diminished control over their lives, residents may turn to worship, prayer, and meditation for comfort and strength. "Whether religious or otherwise, frail elders need an abundance of rituals," she reports. "This underlines the importance of conducting a spiritual assessment and encouraging elders to reflect upon their lives. In particular, people with dementia often respond to what is familiar, so it is vital to explore this with them, if possible, or with family members." Here is another reason to participate in a program like "Honor My Wishes," which we described earlier in the book. It involves managing not only your financial portfolio but your social, psychological, and spiritual affairs as well.

"Even with cognitive decline, we can still communicate soul to soul," Marty affirms. "Wise care providers understand that full mental awareness is not necessary to relate to people. I have even had people with dementia pick up nonverbal signs of stress in my life. Because of the need to adapt to a lack of cognitive skills, they may depend more on nonverbal cues. I've learned from them how to take things more slowly and that nonverbal behavior is infinitely more important. If we are incongruent, they will pick this up. Unfortunately, in many nursing homes, the nonverbal message given to patients reflects a sense of detachment and indifference."

This underscores the necessity of caregivers engaging in their own spiritual work. Especially with people who are cognitively impaired, staff cannot simply put in time performing duties. With dementia, the "quality of the moment" becomes a special imperative. As others have emphasized in this book, it means being attentively present with people. "Whatever we are doing with such a person, whether routine such as turning a body in a bed, the touch and connection at that moment becomes all important," Marty reflects. "To do this, we must examine ourselves, our attitudes, and our fears. In workshops, I often talk about keeping 'heart' in one's work. In Latin, the letters 'COR' mean heart. It is the root of the word 'encouragement.' Ultimately, I believe that no matter what job they have in a caregiving environment, workers must keep heart in their work. It is the work of encouragement with both residents and staff. We must have people who feel called to this work because, especially with dementia, people know in a minute when someone does not have a kind heart."

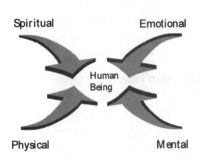

The diagram above represents a way of visualizing Marty's insight. With a frail, cognitively impaired elder, the physical and mental aspects are diminished, but the emotional and spiritual functions remain intact. Caregivers need to explore ways to communicate through these functions. Several of the resources and tools in this book should be of assistance in this respect.

Marty conducts workshops on many topics and offers two educational series especially for congregations. The first class entitled, *Aging: Our Grandparents, Our Parents, Our Own*, addresses the basics of the aging process. She talks about the fear associated with aging, some of the common, false assumptions about the process of growing old, and employs *The Aging I.Q.* published by National Institute on Aging that asks 20 questions testing one's knowledge of aging (http://www.niapublications.org/tipsheets/pdf/Whats_Your_Aging_IQ.pdf).

A second offering, *Toward the Future*, engages participants in thinking about quality of life, building internal and family resources, and finding meaning and purpose as we age. She includes material on creating Ethical Wills (Riemer and Stampfer 1991). The concept evolves from an old Jewish tradition where people going to battle leave a recording of their particular history, values, and beliefs. The task involves leaving your story and your legacy with future generations. Marty informs us, "I ask people to take six pieces of paper to write about the history of their family: (1) opening; (2) the family; (3) religious observances and insights; (4) personal history; (5) ethical ideals and practices; and (6) closing.

People also are encouraged to develop a spiritual autobiography. Briefly, this involves developing a lifeline of significant, spiritual events in your life and then writing about them. What was the situation and why was it significant? What persons were involved and what values emerged? What did you learn and what gifts surfaced? How has this event impacted your life? The process helps us to more concretely state our beliefs about ourselves, about our relationships with others, and about God and/or the universe. Marty recommends *Remembering Your Story: A Guide to Spiritual Autobiography* by Richard L. Morgan as a good resource (Morgan 1996, p. 20).

Somewhat related, Marty shares, "Some years ago at an American Society on Aging conference, Father Richard Sweeney spoke about six basic spiritual tasks of aging. They are:

- To establish a sense of self-worth apart from the externals (don't sweat the small stuff);
- To freely surrender those parts of our lives that we can no longer do, such as giving up driving a car;
- To become a teacher or mentor to others;
- To seek and share wisdom with one another;
- To see life as having meaning and value but not being perfect;
- To face death and afterlife questions.

He saw these as later life tasks that revolve around spirituality. Obviously, not all elders complete these tasks. Some of them find themselves stuck or blocked from being able to progress. There are some grumpy, narrow-minded older adults."

One of Marty's mentors is Jim Gambone, a filmmaker who wrote a book entitled *Refirement: A Guide to Midlife and Beyond,* who asserts that we should view our lives as having purpose and ministry regardless of our age (Gambone 2000). "I participated in a workshop with a number of older adults where we engaged in a refirement ritual. These elders were commissioned to continue their ministry because there is no retirement age for it, to pray, and to keep invested in life. As mentioned earlier, we need to build more of such rituals for elders because they experience many transitions, such as leaving one's home for an assisted living arrangement, giving up the keys to the car, or experiencing the death of a pet."

Marty acknowledges the difficulty elders have with leaving their homes. "Author Kathleen Fischer in a Seattle workshop has described a ritual of saying good-bye to each room and perhaps taking along a small, meaningful object. We need these markers of particular events; they don't have to be particularly religious, but they keep the spirit alive in one way or another."

In a class Marty teaches on social and cultural aspects of aging, she introduces *ethnographic interviewing*, which differs from asking closed-ended questions such as "When and where were you born?" Rather, we ask something like, "Tell me what it was like to live during the depression years." By asking such open-ended questions with elders, the respondent leads the interview. It becomes a way of empowering people and getting to the narrative core of one's life. See the Appendix for additional information.

In discussions with elders, Marty also believes in the importance of addressing the subject of hope. "Not in the sense of promoting unrealistic expectations," she states, "but as having four different aspects. They are:

- Hope for life after death, which is the spiritual dimension;
- Hope as an existential process of how we cope with suffering. How do we make sense out of suffering? What are the lessons learned?
- Hope as a rational thought process whereby people establish goals and pursue the resources to meet those goals, taking control over one's life and over time. Interestingly, this is all part of the care-planning process utilized by professionals.
- Hope as a relational process. It entails how we relate to other people so they have a sense of hope. It includes together maintaining belief in a positive outcome, even if it means a peaceful death."

One question that might be asked to generate hope would be, "What would make a good day for you?" For an example of an answer to this question and to testimony of the nature and power of hope, we recommend the film *Tuesdays With Morrie*, as well as the book, *Morrie: In His Own Words* (Schwartz 1996).

In general, Marty believes that caregivers need to realize that everyone ages in their own way and experiences spirituality differently. "We cannot lay our beliefs upon them. In addition, we must realize that aging people have strengths, and we need to build upon them. People can build upon inner and outer resources. Inner resources might include one's faith and a sense of perseverance. With outer resources, the strength becomes a willingness to ask for help from others. Most elders cherish autonomy. However, self-sufficiency becomes a weakness when we use our power to keep others from helping us when we need assistance.

"Finally, I strongly believe that the spiritual aspect of life is not separate from physical, cognitive, and emotional facets, but is integral to all of them. Wendy Lustbader describes spirituality as the explanation for being alive, as choosing one life plan over another, and as stories about our lives and the lives of others that help us make sense out of our lives (Lustbader & Hooyman 1994, p. 31). Richard Morgan pictures this as three overlapping circles representing 'me', 'you' and 'God.' The best relationships are based upon the co-joining of these three circles and their respective stories" (Morgan 2002, p. 20).

Eastern Thought as It Relates to Soulful Aging

Charles Emlet, PhD, MSW

"I've been thinking about the process of aging for about 30 years, first as an undergraduate student at about the time I began considering social work as a profession," explains Charles Emlet. As an associate professor of Social Work at the University of Washington, Tacoma, he teaches courses on aging in American society and on spirituality and social work practice. Much of his research is focused upon older adults with HIV disease.

"Aging involves many things such as impermanence, fear, death, spirituality, acceptance, and love," believes Dr. Emlet. "Both Hindu and Buddhist traditions acknowledge aging, disease, and death as a part of our human existence. Often they come framed as a function of the transient nature of the human body. Saint Francis referred to his body as 'brother ass,' something that had to be carted around, whereas for him the soul was immortal."

Born in approximately 2500 BC, Buddhism emerged from the shock and despair of young prince Siddartha after learning of disease, old age, and death. Dr. Emlet relates, "A prince in India, which today is Southern Nepal, lived in a compound where nothing was allowed to exist that was not essentially perfect, young, and vibrant. However, being rather inquisitive, Siddartha persuades one of his assistants to lead him out of the compound. Shortly thereafter they meet an old man shakily walking with a staff, representing old age. Next, they encounter a person laying very ill, illustrating disease. Finally, they come across a corpse, depicting death.

"Shocked and despaired by these events, Siddartha left the compound and spent the rest of his life seeking answers to these problems. He eventually sat under a tree where he experienced enlightenment, becoming whom we now know as the Buddha. Buddha's teachings include an understanding the value of *being*."

Dr. Emlet refers us to Ram Dass, a former professor at Stanford and Harvard who in the 1960s left teaching to pursue a spiritual journey. In his book, *Still Here: Embracing Aging, Changing, and Dying,* he writes about retirement anxiety: "After having been applauded [in our culture] for busy-ness and productivity, there is guilt about stillness. This attitude is endemic to our materialistic, youth-oriented culture and counterproductive to our approach to conscious aging, which requires a great deal of stillness in order to awaken to the wisdom within us" (Dass 2000, p. 100).

Often Ram Dass speaks about the contrasting differences between ego and soul. Looking through the lens of the individualistic ego, we seem so caught up in youth, adulthood, production, and consumerism. Aging is ignored (a form of denial), feared, or reframed to reward those in the earlier years of elderhood. With respect to the latter, we bestow awe and honor upon people such as Lou and Jim Whittker who in their mid-seventies climb to the peaks of huge mountains. Unfortunately, we set them up as models for aging, creating unreasonable expectations for most of society. Such examples convey the message that even if we are aging, we should act young and be productive, which certainly creates some interesting conflicts.

For an alternative to this viewpoint, Dr. Emlet makes reference to the ancient Law of Manu that provides some mandates of how we live our lives and the role, place, and purpose of old age in that process. It contains some interesting ideas for us to reflect upon. One text reads: "When the householder sees wrinkles in his skin, grayness in his hair and the sons of his sons, let him retire to the forest, detached from family life."

The Law of Manu expands upon this in the context of the four stages of Hindu life. Each stage has its own discipline geared to develop spiritual consciousness.

I. The first stage is that of the student. Learning becomes the focus, and great importance is given to the development of discipline and purity.
II. The second stage begins around 21 years of age when the person becomes a householder, forming and raising a family, establishing oneself in a career or job, and becoming an active member of the community.
III. Called "vanaprasthia," the third stage begins in the mid-forties and embraces a time of deepening contemplation and the reorientation of desires, motives, and the essential character of one's activities. The profit motive is given up, along with any motivation for personal gain, as a shift occurs toward serving the "Whole" of which he sees himself a part, but without remuneration.
IV. Known as "sannyasa," the fourth stage becomes the renunciation phase. This is the same Sanskrit term used to identify a monk or one who has renounced the world for the spiritual life. This individual becomes an elder who has gained wisdom, who renounces the outer goals of life, and who is no longer partaking in social or political concerns. The end of life is drawing near, and one should make as much spiritual progress as possible. Hindus believe in reincarnation, so the task is to make as much progress as possible to contribute to a better situation the next time around (Tathagatannda 2004; http://www.vedanta-newyork.org/articles/vedanta101_7.htm).

The ideas expressed in these stages, especially the last stage, are quite foreign to our Western thinking of doing, productivity, and "worthiness." Ram Dass says, "We hear the fear of disempowered role-lessness; the fear of having nothing structured, nothing we're 'supposed' to be doing, that becomes so palpable around retirement time. To counteract [their anxiety], people often throw themselves into other activities, such as volunteerism, second families, [unending] vacationing, or hobbies and avocations, [in order] to maintain a sense of having some purpose. Though there is certainly nothing wrong with being busy, the desperation that often prompts these activities does create a shadow" (Dass 2000, pp. 99–100).

"What Ram Dass is attempting to say is that society seems to mandate that we must be busy and productive," Dr. Emlet asserts. "The problem is asking [society] for external validation of value and worth, hoping for an affirmative response.

"But what if we turned this process on its head? What if aging offers us a tremendous opportunity for spiritual growth, to cultivate stillness and wisdom?" Dr. Emlet refers again to Ram Dass, who speaks about his father as he grew older, slowing down, being more focused and attentive to each task, whether it was getting into a car or settling into his favorite armchair. "He found satisfaction in the completion of each small task; he would smile with contentment and say quietly, 'There we are.'" (Dass 2000, p. 206).

As a social worker, Dr. Emlet relates the story of visiting an elderly man who was near death. "It was a memorable visit because the gentleman was so spiritually connected and centered, obviously at the acceptance stage of dying. Not only could I not do anything for him, but when I left the house I remember chuckling to myself that I didn't help him; he helped me. I took so much more away from the experience than anything I gave to him. The man was unable 'to do' anything and yet, by his 'being present' with me, he provided an invaluable service."

Dr. Emlet underscores that acceptance is the final stage of Elisabeth Kubler-Ross's stages of dying. The stages are:

Denial and isolation: In this stage, the person denies that death is really going to take place.
Anger: The dying person realizes that denial can no longer be maintained, and very often, feelings of anger, resentment, rage, and envy follow.
Bargaining: In this phase, the dying person develops the hope that death can somehow be postponed or delayed.
Depression: Here the dying person comes to accept the certainty of death.
Acceptance: The dying person develops a sense of peace; an acceptance of one's fate; and, in many cases, a desire to be left alone (Kubler-Ross 1969).

The last stage of acceptance reminds us of the final, intimate dialogue between Mitch Albom and Morrie Schwartz in the movie version of *Tuesdays With Morrie*. Dying from the debilitating Lou Gehrig's disease, Morrie (played by Jack Lemmon) is visited by his old student, Mitch (played by Hank Azaria), a very busy, "doing" sports writer, who is challenged not only to confront his own mortality but to avoid simply rushing through life without taking the time to be truly present to anything or anyone, including the girlfriend he reportedly loves.

MITCH: What if all of this was just wasted on me?

MORRIE: Do you think that could happen?

MITCH: Out in the world, outside this room, things aren't so clear. . . . What if you just want to run like hell when you see death coming? What if . . . we can't learn it because we're really not like you?

MORRIE: Yes, but you are like me. Everybody is.

MITCH: Nobody's like you. If it took your death to teach me these things, then I'd rather not learn them. All the things you said I'd give back in one minute. I don't want [your death] to happen. . . . What's the point? I just can't accept it. I don't want you to die. I guess I flunked the course.

MORRIE: Death ends a life, not a relationship (*Tuesdays with Morrie* 2001).

Morrie's overall testimony in the video and in the book serves as an excellent example of gerotranscendence. His ego integrity emerges, and self-integration occurs. His interactions tend to have more depth and intimacy. The borders between time and space seem to recede for him. There is an expanded understanding of the connectedness of everything and of exploring interrelationships. Certainly for Morrie, there is a lessening of fear, and the acceptance of death as a transition comes to the forefront.

ARCHITECT OF SACRED SPACE

Jim Fondriest, Pastoral Care/Bereavement Coordinator

The process of dying has been described by some as entering the "dark night of the soul." As the Pastoral Care/Bereavement Coordinator at Hospice of the Cleveland Clinic in Cleveland, Ohio, Jim Fondriest encounters many hospice patients and confirms this perception. He affirms, "It is indeed a dark night, but it is also an invitation and a journey. It often reminds me of the pain of childbirth. It's not pretty. But it is okay to go there, and those of us in hospice provide people with the sacred space for this process to occur. As chaplains, we call ourselves spiritual care providers. We don't fix things, but create the space for people to do their own work. In a sense, we are really architects."

According to Jim, a study conducted by the American Society on Aging affirms that aging is much more than a biological phenomenon; it includes social, psychological, and spiritual dimensions. "To grow old often involves becoming more aware of who we are," he asserts. "As we age, we begin to strip away an identity we attached to ourselves during earlier years. Back then, we defined ourselves essentially by our association with our roles related to family, career, religion, ethnic origins, and the like. However, as we move into elderhood, often we begin to disassociate from many of these responsibilities and relationships. The spiritual terminology associated with it is *The Via Negativa*, befriending darkness, letting go and letting be [Fox 1983]. As we move closer to death, some elders ask existential questions like, 'Who am I, really?' However, no final answer comes to light. Rather it is more of an ongoing quest and a journey."

In the late 1970s Jim worked in Escondido, California, with Elisabeth Kubler-Ross, renowned for her exploration of the process of grieving. "She conducted the grief workshops, and my job involved taking people up a mountain at the end of the week to engage in a ritual of letting go of the grief," he informs us. "We would build a fire, and people would write down their grief issues and attach them to pine cones, then throw them in the flames. This was followed with a meal of bread and wine.

"Kubler-Ross used to say that we are born with only two natural fears—fear of falling and fear of loud noise. We learn all other fears from our parents and other significant adults in our lives. Also, our Western culture promotes certain types of fear. For example, we are taught to live in the past or in the future as a way of coping with worry and fright, which seriously detracts from living in the precious present. Much of what we fear becomes associated with pain. In particular, hospice performs a wonderful service in terms of alleviating physical pain. However, we need to face emotional and spiritual pain head-on, for it is the only arena through which we can heal and grow. What we do as chaplains in spiritual care involves helping people to face the pain, not attempting to remove it from them."

Jim believes that most terminal patients are able to deal with their issues, especially if they have been served by hospice for a period longer than a few days or weeks. There exists a phenomenon called *terminal restlessness*. People may slip into a coma and become very agitated. Terminal restlessness is a syndrome observed in patients in their last days of life. It is a variant of delirium and refers to a spectrum of signs of central nervous system irritability that may include restlessness, agitation, distressed vocalizing, twitching, jerking, or recurrent movements. Many causes have been suggested for this restlessness, but certainly one of them centers upon unresolved spiritual and relationship issues. Jim believes that people often enter deeply into the psyche or soul, dealing with matters that must be confronted. On the other hand, some people face an issue consciously, name it, speak about it, and grow through it. Another word describing this process is *forgiveness*, a word in scripture literally meaning "to lift up, let go and send away."

"Unfortunately, toward the end of their journey, the dying aren't always able to come back to tell you about it," Jim reports. "However, returning in one form or another is part of the journey. To return involves entering a time of transformation, rebirth, and celebration."

Like the ritual of taking people up a mountain to release their grief, Jim performs many other rituals with patients. One of his patients in her early fifties was, like Jim, a Roman Catholic, and she requested that he offer her communion. "During another visit, the woman asked me to read a portion of her journal," he remembers. "She said that she wanted me to conduct her funeral and therefore wanted me to get to know her more intimately. I was deeply moved by the journal entries and especially by one of her reflections: 'Hope is not the conviction that all will turn out well, but that all will be well no matter how it turns out.' After reading the journal, we began the ritual of actually preparing her funeral service."

The Hospice of the Cleveland Clinic also has a residential unit, and Jim serves it as well. One of the rituals for the staff involves washing a person's body upon death and anointing it with oil in preparation for burial. This connects to the story of Jesus's anointment and burial following his death.

The value of rituals, Jim believes, lies in their ability to lead us in the direction of the sacred. They often contribute to the challenge of getting away from analytical, thinking processes and going deep within oneself. Especially in the West, we are such compulsive thinkers. He recounts, "Someone once said that desire is the source of all suffering. Basically, it means that the things to which we are most attached cause us the greatest grief. So, if we are attached to some occurrence in the past, it will continue to haunt us and cause pain. Or, we may be attached to an expectation or hope for the future. That creates suffering in the sense that we may remain in a difficult relationship, place, or job hoping that one of these days, things will get better."

When a patient enters hospice, the entire family becomes the focus of a plan of care. The staff helps them process what is occurring and provides a significant amount of education. The staff often leads people through a life review progression using material from experts like Ira Byock, MD, past president of the American Palliative Association. His book, *Dying Well,* outlines five simple phrases that largely contribute to facilitating a good death (Byock 1997). They are:

> Please forgive me;
> I forgive you;
> I love you;
> Thank you; and
> Good-bye.

Dr. Byock also reclaims the traditional meaning of "good-bye" as "God be with you," a blessing that we all can use, whether parting from someone for an hour, a day, or at the end of a lifetime.

Similar end-of-life tasks identified by hospice social worker Dee Caplan-Tuke, include:

> Taking care of business;
> Arriving at a sense of completion in terms of community relations;
> Having a sense of the meaning of one's life;
> Loving and forgiving oneself;
> Experiencing the love of others; and
> Accepting the finality of life.

Jim takes this process one step further, believing that it is important to begin it now, not just wait until the end of life is near. His conviction is supported by a number of prominent philosophers and teachers:

- When Plato was asked at the very end of his life to sum up his whole life's work and his philosophy, he said simply, "Practice dying."
- Leonardo Da Vinci once said, "While I thought I was learning how to live, I was really learning how to die."
- Seneca stated, "Throughout the whole of life, one must continue to learn how to live, and what will amaze you even more, throughout life one must learn how to die."

▮ Jesus taught us to pray, "Thy will be done." This becomes a prayer of surrender and release, an acceptance of "what is" as it relates to life tasks and not simply end-of-life tasks.

In any case, in working with the dying, Jim states, "While maintaining boundaries and not taking on someone's emotional pain, we provide a lot of affirmation and validation of their feelings. I like to speak not about what is a good death, but what is the good in dying. The dark night of the soul is about spiritual suffering and someone coming to a point of surrender. Surrendering means no longer resisting what 'is'; it is letting go of negativity, not mentally labeling things, and ultimately living in the present moment."

Jim maintains that one of our most important challenges of aging holistically involves claiming and expanding our identities. He asserts, "A difference exists between one's life situation and one's life. One's life situation at any given time may be wonderful or horrible, but one's life is always good. This perception comes from dismantling the ego and living in the moment, knowing that to just live and enjoy the moment is enough."

His comments remind us of a delightful book by David Steindl-Rast, *Gratefulness, The Heart of Prayer: An Approach to Life in Fullness*. A Benedictine monk, he states that the path to a life of fullness is to, "Wake up!" It is "to bless whatever there is [before us at the moment], and for no other reason but simply because it is, that is what we are made for as human beings" (Steindl-Rast 1984). In this respect, we might say that one of the essential tasks of elderhood is to be wide awake, to widen our capacity for gratefulness, and, as Jim believes, to simply live in the precious present. Paraphrasing William James describing spirituality as the attempt to be in harmony with the seen and unseen order of things, Jim states, "Spirituality includes being in a right relationship with God, with the world, with the people we care about, and even with the people we don't care about. It's all about writing the music of our own lives."

References

Buber, M. 1923. *I and Thou*. New York: Touchstone 1996 edition.
Byock, I. 1997. *Dying Well: Peace and Possibilities at the End of Life*. New York: Riverside Books.
Dass, R. 2000. *Still Here: Embracing Aging, Changing, and Dying*. NY: Riverside Books.
Fox, M. 1983. *Original Blessing*. Santa Fe, NM: Bear and Co.
Gambone, J. 2000. *Refirement: A Guide to Midlife and Beyond*. Minneapolis, MN: Kirk House Publishers.
Hillman, J. 1996. *The Soul's Code*. New York: Random House.
Kastenbaum, K. 2004. *Death, Society, and Human Experience*. Boston: Pearson Education, Inc.

Kubler-Ross, E. 1969. *On Death and Dying*. New York: Touchstone.

Levoy, G. 1997. *Callings: Finding and Following an Authentic Life*. New York: Harmony Books.

Lustbader, W. and N. Hooyman. 1994. *Taking Care of Aging Family Members: A Practical Guide*. New York: Free Press.

Morgan, R. 1996. *Remembering Your Story: A Guide to Spiritual Autobiography*. Nashville: Upper Room Books.

Palmer, P. 1999. *Let Your Life Speak*. San Francisco: Jossey-Bass.

Riemer, J. and N. Stampfer. 1991. *So That Your Values Live On: Ethical Wills and How to Prepare Them*. Woodstock, VT: Jewish Lights Publishing.

Schwartz, M. 1996. *Morrie: In His Own Words*. New York: Delta.

Steindl-Rast, D. 1984. *Gratefulness, the Heart of Prayer: An Approach to Life in Fullness*. Ramsey, NJ: Paulist Press.

Tathagatannda, S. 2004. *Four Stages of Life*. New York: Vedanta Society of New York. http://www.vedanta-newyork.org/articles/vedanta101_7.htm (accessed July 30, 2006).

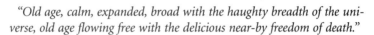

Section 6
Wide-Ranging Innovative Resources and Testimonies

"Old age, calm, expanded, broad with the haughty breadth of the universe, old age flowing free with the delicious near-by freedom of death."

—Edith Wharton
(1862–1937)

In This Section . . . Many eldercare providers bring to the profession a wide range of innovative resources, just a few being music, art, Healing Touch, and life review therapies. In the process, they find themselves blessed by the many intangible gifts they receive in return from elders.

COMMUNICATING AND RESOLVING CONFLICT IN ELDER FAMILY SYSTEMS

John Gibson, DSW, PhD, MSW, MS

John Gibson often punctuates his conversations with elders and their families with stories that speak to a specific situation. As a gerontologist with over 25 years of counseling and coaching experience, he often works with individuals who are facing complex challenges, especially those involving strong emotion, conflict, and pressure.

During the course of interviewing for this book, a number of professional caregivers expressed frustration about gaining agreement from their own elder family members regarding the need for extended care, necessitating leaving their home and entering a long-term care facility. "One of the things I almost always talk about," John says, "is to remind families that most sons and daughters in their fifties and sixties were raised in classrooms where we learned about 'The Little Engine That Could' [Piper 1976]. The little engine says, 'I think I can, I think I can, I know I can, I know I can, I did, I did, I did.' We are also programmed by such phrases as 'Where there's a will, there's a way.' Consequently, we tend to allow these messages to guide our expectations, leading to what we think we *should* be able to accomplish with our aging parents. However, in eldercare, we must be aware that many situations exist where we will fail to achieve what we can imagine as possible. And yet, we have done our best, given the resources available, our parents' compliance, and our limited time and energy."

Essentially, such messages distort the *doing* or thinking energy depicted in Section 1 and are further exacerbated by such popular assertions as Vince Lombardi's "Winning Isn't Everything, It's the Only Thing." For many people, and even more so for elders, such messages often set us up for failure and a huge guilt trip. Overextended, they may lead to fierce competition and to winning at all costs, neither of which is a common attribute of mature elders.

Elders themselves may fall victim to unrealistic expectations. Many experienced challenging situations as children or as young adults, perhaps because of the Great Depression or World War II, John maintains. "They learned to do what I call 'lock on, lock out.' Having endured a depression, they may lock on to a position of surviving anything, no matter what it is, even if there is property loss or some other tragedy happens. In addition, they tend to lock out any doubts they may have of achieving their goal, as well [as experiencing] other people's skepticism, which can result in tremendous stress and potential blindness to reality. Elders who have locked on to an image created by earlier experiences are less flexible and adaptable to their current reality."

John's comments bring to mind our understanding of "moderate risk." If a person enjoys a 95% possibility of succeeding in achieving a goal, there is hardly any risk at all involved in the endeavor. On the other hand, if there is a huge probability of failure, perhaps upwards to 95%, the possibility of disappointment skyrockets. Moderate risk represents a 50%–50% chance of success or failure, wherein our personal efforts and the support of others can make a positive difference in achieving an acceptable outcome. Although many elders may not respond favorably to logic, it may be worth engaging this strategy.

In light of "lock on, lock out," one of John's activities in working with older adults involves beginning in advance to start planting seeds suggesting alternatives. He may ask elders to observe other relatives or neighbors making decisions based upon deteriorating circumstances. He encourages people to talk and to "wonder out loud." "I wonder who paid their bills while they were in the hospital," or, "I wonder if she had any contingency plans in place when she fell and broke her hip." In this manner, questions can be raised about certain situations, not about the individual personally, but about a third party. This approach involves elders in potential-problem solving and in exploring "what-if" scenarios based upon other people's experiences.

John counsels care providers to avoid arguments and to explore alternatives, using this approach. For example, reflecting upon, "Yes, Uncle John had a bad experience rehabilitating in that nursing home. But, I wonder how it is going for your friend Betty? Have you been in contact with her?" Again, it is planting seeds that expand choices.

"Also related to this strategy is to begin exploring planning criteria," John underscores. "For example, if one of the neighbors entered a retirement home, you might ask an elder to speculate on how such a decision was made based upon that person's wishes and needs. How did she/he decide it was time to make this move? How might examining some options ahead of time be beneficial? The discussion might proceed something like, 'Dad, while you're still driving, perhaps you could take your car to the new facility with you; you would still be able to drive around town and even take some of your new friends with you.'"

John describes this as life-contingency planning akin to creating a will and preparing for the circumstances surrounding one's death. The BenefitsCheckUp offered through the National Council on Aging could serve as a starting point for discussions. In addition, as mentioned earlier, the list of questions and ratings designed to measure the quality of nursing homes, developed by Marilyn Rantz and The Quality Improvement Program for Missouri, may serve to stimulate discussions and expand alternatives (Rantz, Zwygart-Stauffacher, & Flesner 2005; www.nursinghomehelp.org/OIQ.pdf). John likens the experience to creating a mental map of alternatives.

As a way of communicating appropriate choices, John may tell stories of other clients who have faced similar issues and describe how their decisions were made and impacted them. John believes that using stories and talking about a third party lessons the opportunity for elders to become defensive.

There are many times, however, when there is little or no time to plant seeds or to engage in contingency planning. "First," John responds, "I would attempt to find out what they most deeply value. As an illustration, if one of the things they value relates to not being a burden on anyone, then this provides a point of leverage to explore how might this person become a burden. I will create a story first so the elder doesn't simply 'lock out,' such as, 'In Joe's situation, it turned out, much to his surprise, that he would be less of a burden by moving to an extended care facility and would have more choices than if he remained at home.' The story taps into the elder's value system.

"Another technique relates to using an emotional plea as opposed to using reason. A son or daughter might say, 'I know you don't believe you need someone to come into the house a few hours each day, but I worry and I know it's my problem. For my peace of mind, it would be a tremendous gift if you would try this for a period of time.' Unfortunately, it may appear as a personal rebuff if the personal request is turned down, which illustrates one reason why care providers often recommend sticking to reason and logic rather than appealing for personal consideration."

What we often experience in such situations entails parent-child role reversal, notes John. Therefore, as difficult as it may be, the family member must give him- or herself permission to set boundaries, remembering that we are responsible *to* but not *for* another person. At this point in the conflict, if the elder is almost totally uncooperative, unwilling to collaborate or compromise in coming forward with a solution, the only two options may be to "give-in" and let the chips fall where they may, or to adopt an assertive position, such as, "Well, this is your choice, but I will only be available to visit you twice each week."

Here, John suggests a discussion such as, "Let me share my crystal ball with you, and admittedly it is foggy, but it projects the possibility that you may injure yourself at home and have no way to get help for a period of time. It could also result in being hospitalized and then entering a period of rehabilitation in a nursing home. But, as we have discussed, another option is to enter an assisted living residence where you will be much less likely to harm yourself. Also, you can meet new friends and be able to come and go as you wish." Again, the focus is upon choice and consequence. In the situation of assisted living as an alternative, the recommended approach involves holding up a positive image and reinforcing it again and again. Sometimes John even asks if an elder would care to work with him in developing a list of positive consequences, leaving it with the client if desired.

Fear tends to be the underlying emotion behind "locked in" behaviors, such as the determination to remain living at home. Knowing this and understanding basic values, how then can the care provider explore imaginative ways to find how values can be honored and fear diminished in a new and different setting? How can what is important to the elder be taken with him or her to a new environment? One such innovative strategy would be to take pictures of one's home for inclusion in a memory book or, as an even better alternative, to invite the elder to take a trip throughout the home accompanied by a video camera. This could become a historical document to be shared with relatives and with new friends in a new setting that can become a part of one's life review process.

We could also assist the elder to make a new home out of an apartment in an assisted living environment. All activities like this work to build a bridge from the old environment into the new setting. However, keep in mind that there needs to be a time of preparation so the older person doesn't view it as a too-quick solution. Adequate life review time needs to be incorporated into the process.

In addition, be aware that family dynamics often shift when a crisis arises, John explains, noting that illness changes the family member who is ill and that the adult children in a family experienced different childhoods. And, he relates, "Often conflicting feelings arise among family members that are incompatible. For instance, with a cancer diagnosis, one feeling may be the desire of family members to do whatever is possible to help restore health, which may be in conflict with the fear of financial loss. Or, negative feelings may come into play because of time pressures relative to work and to other family needs, bringing on resentment caused by the need for increased caregiving. Such feelings can bring on anger, shame, and guilt. This can make it quite difficult for a group of family members to make appropriate decisions and may lead to the vital need to solicit the support of a professional facilitator to help the family sort through complex issues and feelings and make decisions."

If the theory of gerotranscendence is viable, which maintains that all elders contain at least a seed of wanting to have meaning in the autumn of their lives, then it becomes imperative to build upon this research. John believes the best way to accomplish this would involve, whenever possible, building upon the stories of other elders who successfully transitioned into older age maturity. Some practical guidelines for applying gerotranscendence are shared below (Tornstam 2005, pp. 131–84).

- Whenever possible, reduce preoccupation with the body and matters of health.
- Encourage the sharing of stories about pleasant experiences and how they may have contributed to personal growth. Seek out instances when challenges were met and problems were solved.
- Encourage talk about legacy, i.e., "What accomplishments in your life are you proud of, ones that made a positive difference in the lives of others?"
- Ask the elder to describe an ideal day in her/his life as a way of uncovering values.
- Encourage small choices as well as the big ones, i.e., "Where would you like me to place these flowers?" or "Where shall we go for a drive today?"
- Whenever appropriate, ask for opinions, advice, and counsel about family, cultural, or world situations (soliciting the wisdom coming from the elder's many life experiences).

- Describe and seek out interest in holistic therapies, e.g., massage, music, art, meditation, yoga, etc.
- Seek out opportunities to talk about people who have died and about death.
- Use adult-appropriate language and images as opposed to treating an elder as a child.
- Engage and encourage humor and laughter.
- Encourage reading books and watching movies that uplift, honor, and respect elders.

Caring for the Wise Ones

Michelle Bowman, RN

When Longmont Memorial Hospital, Longmont, Colorado, decided to develop an outpatient senior wellness program in 1991, it seemed a natural choice to appoint Michelle Bowman as its program manager. With her passion for elders and her geriatric experience, she acknowledges, "It became a wonderful opportunity, because I was given a clean palette to develop the whole program."

Michelle began the program by extensive researching and benchmarking, after which she approached a number of the hospital's doctors, asking them to identify their favorite older adult patients. She developed a list of contacts she calls "the wise ones" and, one by one, invited them to participate in a ten-person advisory committee. She said to them, "You have much more life experience than I have, so tell me what you would like to see made available in the wellness program."

Named PrestigePLUS, the center represents a prestigious time of life and is inspired by nursing homes in China that are called "homes for respecting the elderly." With a total of 27 employees under her supervision, she also manages the Department of Complementary Care at the hospital. Funding comes from insurance payments, private pay, and through a foundation that provides scholarships.

Michelle's enthusiasm bears witness to a passion for working with "the wise ones," and she views it as her life's work and bliss. She began her career as an ICU nurse and during her first summer was involved in 13 cardiopulmonary resuscitations and deaths. This difficult experience led her to work in a telemetry step-down unit instead of the ICU, where there were large numbers of older patients. Subsequently, she chaired the hospital's task force on aging. "I've always had an affinity toward older people, even as a little girl," she recalls.

Michelle views a "wise one" as a person who is older than she and who has more life experiences. In addition, taking some insights from Rabbi Zalman Schachter-Shalomi, founder of the Spiritual Eldering Institute, a "wise one" is someone who has the ability to purposely share and apply knowledge and experience with common sense and insight. As we age, consciousness expands. For example, Michelle tells us of the 80-year-old woman who spoke of her deceased husband, reporting, "You know, if I was living in this current culture, I would divorce my husband, because I was miserable with him my whole life. I stayed in the marriage because that was what I was supposed to do. Now that he's dead, I'm having fun."

"We started the senior program by offering a variety of conventional topics," Michelle relates. "But after a year it became rather boring, and I was told that if we offered another session on hypertension they were going to vomit," she recalls laughing. The advisory board informed Michelle that they wanted the hospital to swim further upstream and to offer more holistic options. They wanted programs they had heard about in other cultures. "So, because of the 'wise ones' on the board, we decided to conduct a mini-survey," she relates. "We determined that, even in our little community of Longmont, people were involved in some complementary and alternative medicine (CAM) healing practices. When the data was presented to the hospital, they initially did not want to travel down this road because of the risk and the possibility of a backlash. Undeterred, the 'wise ones' decided to conduct a fundraiser for the purposes of providing additional education by sending me to China. So in 1994, I went to China with the American Society on Aging. I was one of 20 delegates who spent a month exploring Eastern medicine and healing modalities."

Upon Michelle's return, the first T'ai Chi class was formed. For those unfamiliar with this modality, T'ai Chi is an exercise involving movements of the body done in coordination with the mind and with one's respiration. Some people describe it as a practice of flowing clouds and streams, or like pulling thread from a cocoon. Simply put, it involves coordinating oneself with the fundamental healing energies of the universe. Illustrating its impact, Michelle tells the story of one participating woman who had lost four inches in height from degenerative arthritis and osteoporosis and was losing 2-4% of her bone density per year. "Betty Stewart was 84 at the time and today is in her nineties. Up until recently, she participated in the long form of T'ai Chi daily. She eventually gained back height and experienced an increase in her bone density," Michelle explains happily. "Designed to introduce it to others, Betty even joined our traveling T'ai Chi team and has developed a modified form of the discipline and introduced it to elders younger than herself in a local residential facility, many of whom were in a wheelchair or unable to walk."

Trained in acupuncture, Michelle administered her first treatment to Betty when she was 90 years old. "I felt that I was putting needles into someone who was pure spirit," she recalls. "After visiting with her the first time, I came home and wept. It wasn't out of sadness, but because it felt like something way beyond human physical experience. It touched the deepest part of my core. When the needles were in place, Betty confided a very personal, traumatic situation, something she had never told anyone in her entire life. I knew that I had deeply touched something that allowed her to reveal an extremely personal experience."

With 14 massage therapists on staff, a number of other healing massage modalities offered at the center include cranial-sacral massage, deep tissue massage, Swedish hot stone massage, and manual lymph drainage. The latter is used in mainstream Europe with people who have had lymph node dissection, notes Michelle. It opens the lymphatic system and reduces swelling. The center offers 400–450 massages per month in the outpatient clinic, totaling overall about 8,000 visits per year. Seventy percent of the client base is over age 60.

Today, the program also enlists eight acupuncturists, all employees of the hospital. The staff includes two Chinese herbalists, one from China and a Western herbalist who enjoys a statewide reputation. In addition, they provide a wide variety of other therapies including Healing Touch, Reiki, and music therapy.

Continuing Michelle says, "We have reminiscing classes at the center. We have a personal staff historian who assists in the process. She is a 'crone' in the highest sense of that word, an honored elder who serves as a facilitator. She also conducts the entire end-of-life planning classes. We've done 'writing your life' classes and have actually published books about people's lives. We believe storytelling represents the key to people's health. When people share their stories, healing becomes automatic."

Believing strongly in synchronicity and the connectivity of all things, Michelle shares the amazing story of her visit to the home of a very dear 92-year-old friend where she happened to observe a number of cruise ship brochures laying on the table. Her friend, Irene, abruptly informed Michelle that the two of them were going on a cruise together. She said, "Maybe if I take you on a cruise to find you a new husband, I can leave this planet. You know I'm ready to pass on. Besides, I booked and paid for us on an arthritis association cruise; you will be speaking to the group about Chinese medicine." Amazing as it sounded at the time, the two friends subsequently went on the cruise ship, which docked at St. Croix. There they were met by Jon Bowman, whereupon Irene said, "That's him! I told you we would find you a new husband." Michelle and Jon were married four months later.

Later, Irene waited to die until Michelle and her husband had a baby girl. "Irene was cosmically connected," Michelle believes, "and taking me on the cruise to find my husband represented one of the last pieces of work she was to perform on this planet."

Michelle practices active imagination quite frequently and envisions having a council of "wise ones" assisting her from the other side of this life, elders who have been served by the wellness center and who have subsequently passed on. She still speaks to Irene, along with a host of other prestigious friends who have crossed over.

Some may view this as being weird, but it correlates with quantum physics' perception of time and space as being not linear but circular and with the observation of the universe as being multidimensional. In *Leaves of Grass*, Walt Whitman supports this observation, saying, "I do not think seventy years is the time of a man or woman, nor that seventy million years is the time of man or woman, nor that years will ever stop the existence of me, or anyone else." Active imagination is really a relatively new expression of one of the oldest forms of prayer and meditation.

According to Michelle, a new program was recently developed at the Center entitled, *How Will My Story End?* Unlike eager readers who can skip ahead to determine how a story ends, we cannot shape our final days. However, we can begin to celebrate and honor our lives and gain a better understanding over our destiny by asking certain questions. How do you define quality of life? What is a good death? What has been the meaning of your life? What loose ends need to be addressed? Participants in this program are invited to read books associated with *The Heart of the Matter: Literature, Medicine and Values,* a reading and movie discussion curriculum that offers the opportunity to gain a greater understanding of the ethical issues in medical care and end-of-life concerns. The program also encourages reflection and discussion of medical ethics issues in contemporary life. The Colorado Endowment for the Humanities has assembled a list of novels, plays, and stories that ask such important questions and offer new insights.

One of the books (also a movie) is *Whose Life Is It Anyway?,* by Brian Clark, in which Ken Harrison, a central character, survives a terrible car accident that leaves him paralyzed. When he decides that he wants life-saving dialysis discontinued so he can die on his own terms, his decision precipitates a medical, ethical, and legal conflict between physicians devoted to the practice of paternalistic, aggressive treatment (Clark 1978). Inspired by the consumer rights movement, the dramatic action of this play focuses upon the issue commonly known as the "right to die," an individual's right to refuse medical treatment.

Another beautiful film about end of life is *Wit*, based upon a play by Margaret Edson, in which Vivian Bearing becomes a hard-nosed professor who has terminal ovarian cancer. As she approaches death, she reflects upon the cycle of her cancer, the treatments, and significant events in her life. "Few people talk about such things in our culture," Michelle exclaims. "We don't talk about death very openly. I struggle with it myself because I fall in love with some of these older 'wise ones' and then they leave; I grieve deeply." It's no wonder! An African proverb states that when an elder dies it is like closing a library.

A few years ago, Michelle was in a car accident and experienced a head injury that impacted her memory. This event caused her to reflect upon what she wanted to do for the rest of her life. Looking forward into the future, Michelle and her husband plan to move to Mexico where they are building a resort in a little village inhabited by many retirees. "The accident moved me to arrive at a sense of calling to Mexico where there are more than one million U.S. retirees," she states. "The environment there is quite conducive to holistic learning, to connecting with nature, and to sharing personal stories, [all of] which represent one of the essential aspects of healing and aging well."

OPTIMISTIC RAINBOW MAKER

Donna Oiland, Community Outreach Coordinator

"Heroes are people who are making rainbows, making the world a better place," affirms Donna Oiland, Community Outreach Coordinator in the Department of Spiritual Care at Evergreen Health Care, Kirkland, Washington. "My husband, who died in 1997, was one of my heroes," she adds. "I love discerning rainbows, seeing the goodness of God in everything," she adds. "My husband was also like that; in fact, in one of his letters to us, he wrote 'Never not do something because I'm not here.' The day he passed away, people marveled that my son and I attended a sports awards assembly, but my husband would have wanted that."

Donna's optimism is even more awesome in that not only did her husband struggle with colon cancer for seven years, but also her daughter died in 2000 and she gained custody of her grandson and is raising him. However, characteristically she remarks, "My grandson is seven years old and it's like I'm working toward a college degree because he is teaching me so much," she laughs. "He's a great guy!"

Much of Donna's work evolves around public speaking, which spans more than 30 years. Today, the focus is on caregiving, especially to the elderly and their families. Interestingly, although not a nurse, she completed a parish nursing course, which she believes helps people focus on seeing people as more than just a body. It means being an advocate. She also received training as hospice volunteer, as well as to be a Stephen minister, a transdenominational Christian education ministry that provides high-quality training and resources to strengthen and expand lay ministry in congregations.

Community Outreach's mission involves opening conversations with people and increasing sensitivity around end-of-life issues. It includes giving people approaching the end of their lives appropriate tools and insights, as well as encouraging them to see themselves as a collection of wisdom. Their lives may be on a downward spiral, but they still have much to give.

It encompasses training and support for caregivers, Donna informs us. "I conduct a variety of workshops, including topics such as spirituality and aging and a program entitled *Let's Talk About Dying*. When we first considered offering this workshop on dying, we questioned whether anyone would participate. However, 90 people attended the first event and 125 came to a second one. During the workshop, we encourage people to engage in conversations before a crisis arises. The average age of participants ranges from people in their twenties to elders.

"There is a huge number of people in the 'sandwich generation' who may need to take care of both their children and elderly parents. They want to know how to prepare for the storm, or now that they face the storm, what kinds of things they need to do."

We perceive a twofold task in this respect. The first involves taking care of tangible needs, such as planning for a funeral and for the disposal of property if there is no surviving spouse. The second aspect focuses upon emotional and spiritual issues. Donna believes that the latter is just as, if not more, important because if people work through the intangible issues, the rest will follow. "But, I'm not sure we can do much of the emotional work until toward the end of one's life when we know that death is in the near future," she reflects. "I am reminded of something Elisabeth Kubler-Ross said, that our finiteness is a friend who walks beside us. That friend provides meaning to the life by helping us to accept the fact that we will not live forever. If we can accept this friend as a gift and companion, we can then value the time that is left to us."

"My husband," Donna tells us, "is a wonderful example of someone who had a 'good death.' He was 50 years old and, as I said, lived with colon cancer for seven years. I continue to view him as an amazing man, especially when it came down to facing death. Loving his family occupied the last eight months of his life. He wrote us letters, prepared a notebook, and even prepared the eulogy for his memorial service. I didn't know he had done this until just before he died. He asked a friend to read it. It began by welcoming people to his service and by thanking them for coming. Then he said that I objected to his writing the eulogy (I didn't), but he said, 'She finally threw up her hands and said, well, it's your funeral.' What a gift he gave us. He wasn't present, but he was making us laugh and was taking care of us."

Contrary to the many people who reject their aging, Donna is enjoying growing older. For one thing, she worries less about what people think about her. "My priorities have changed a lot. For example, I used to spend time worrying about what people would think when they entered my home. But, I really don't care anymore. My grandson and I doing silly things like wearing red, rubber noses when we are sitting in the car in traffic," she grins. "We roll the windows down and blow bubbles! Neither of us cares what people think about us."

Continuing she says, "My husband taught me a lot about life when he was dying of cancer. Our relationship with God and our family became the most important things, and after that, nothing else really ever matters."

One of Donna's popular community workshops is on the healing power of laughter and the importance of putting more humor into one's life. "I went through a really challenging time in my life, losing both my husband and daughter," she explains. "Then I read an article about a world laughter tour. It was a very expensive class, but

I decided that I needed to attend. After that, I became certified as a laugh leader. The founder of the movement, Dr. Madan Kataria, a physician in India, observed that his patients were very serious. He was aware of the physical benefits of laughter and invited some patients to a session where he encouraged them to 'laugh for no reason,' which is also the name of his book" (Kataria 2002).

Today a considerable amount of research is being conducted on the health benefits of laughter. Laughter helps to remove the effects of stress and gives the immune system a boost, a critical key for maintaining good health.

According to Donna, children can laugh hundreds of times each day, but when we grow up we often find ourselves pressured to be serious, so we may laugh no more than five to ten times a day. "Our sense of humor is getting sick, and it negatively affects our physical body."

Donna relates, "After taking the laughter class, someone suggested that I offer a workshop on the subject. At first I wasn't very comfortable doing it because I'm not that funny myself, but we announced the workshop in a newsletter and the classroom filled up. It's a matter of being intentional about it. Anyone can laugh without hearing or telling jokes. There are Ho-Ho and Ha-Ha exercises and all kinds of techniques such as hearty laughter, silent laughter, and gallows laughter. I believe laughter represents a form of caring for one's spirit in a very positive manner."

Another major emphasis in Donna's work involves encouraging people to write about and share their stories. "It is very much caring for one's spirit as well. In fact, I believe that people can rewrite their stories. With time, people can stand back and view stressful periods and hardships in a different way. By this I mean viewing a particular event or situation as a gift or challenge. Out of tragic events often evolve new knowledge and skills, which may impact one's future in a very positive and passionate way. From tragedy can come joy."

We thoroughly concur with Donna's viewpoint. For example, when Jim worked as a career specialist for a Seattle-based bank, he had a discussion with a 20-year-old bank teller who claimed that one of her key skills was counseling, even though she had no formal training. She told him about receiving trauma counseling after being raped as a teenager. While working in a financial center, she was robbed twice, again receiving trauma counseling. She became so interested in the discipline that she began volunteering her services to help other trauma victims.

Continuing, Donna says, "I am currently reading a book entitled, *The Gift of Pain* [Brand & Yancey 1997]. I have learned from my own experience that tragedy, challenges, struggles, and pain contribute toward our growing up. The task involves embracing difficulty, not wallowing in it, but reflecting upon what is learned from it and how it has changed our lives. It becomes a huge gift that we give to ourselves. The last seven years have been very difficult for me, but I never want to return to the person I was before this time. My priorities were off base back then; my personal faith grew immensely. So I say, 'Bring it on.'"

Donna believes in the incredible experience of listening to the stories of elders. "If you can hear," she says, "you can listen. They are so fascinating that I don't want to miss anything. I sit with elders in a group and listen to one person's story building upon another's, to the extent that people begin to develop a communal relationship."

"For example," Donna relates, "in one of the story circles I have been facilitating, there is a woman who is about 84. She was an actress who eventually became a part of the Special Forces during World War II. She acted in plays for the armed forces in Europe where she met her future husband, who was an English professor. They separated and divorced when she was 50 years old. Subsequently, she decided to change her name from Dottie to Romney."

Donna enjoys audiotaping someone's story, transcribing it, and handing it back to the individual to read. Often, reading one's story on paper is eye-opening because often people maintain that their life is essentially dull and uneventful. However, upon reading their story and reflecting upon it, they suddenly become awed by the drama-filled events of their lives.

In line with her love for making rainbows, we believe Donna's passion is that of an intense optimist, whose work is congruent with her life's calling. Her work bears testimony to the words of Joseph Campbell, "Follow your bliss and don't be afraid, and doors will open where you didn't know they were going to be" (Campbell 1988).

Life Review, Repair, and Purpose

Julia Balzer Riley, RN, MN, AHN-BC, CET®

Julia Balzer Riley's interest in working with elders was serendipitous. A retired nurse friend introduced her to the work of Rabbi Zalman Schachter-Shalomi (often called Reb Zalman), author of *From Age-ing to Sage-ing* (Schachter-Shalomi 1995). "Sage-ing® is a wellness model for vital, successful aging, redefining what it means to grow older and to harvest the fruit's of one's life work. We both decided to become Certified Sage-ing® Leaders," she recalls. "My passion is reaching out and introducing the leading edge of the baby boomers to proactive aging."

When Reb Zalman turned 60, he found himself overwhelmed by a deep depression stemming from fear of old age. Unable to shake this dark night of the soul, he retreated to the mountains of New Mexico in search of answers. After considerable reflection, meditation, and praying, he began to reject cultural images of old age as a time of loss and detachment, reframing it into a time of joy, living a life of meaning, and mentoring younger generations.

Julia is president and founder of Constant Source Seminars©. She is a certified advanced practice holistic nurse with considerable experience in a broad range of disciplines during the past 40 years of her career. She states that her personal mission is "to respirit, reinspire, and revitalize healthcare providers to deliver sensitive care and find joy and humor and meaning along the journey." She also facilitates expressive arts at the Hospice of Southwest Florida in Sarasota as a Certified Expressive Therapist®.

Julia views her work in spiritual eldering as a twofold process. Life review and life repair represent the first part of the process. The philosopher Soren Kierkegaard reminds us that life can only be understood backwards. Life review involves looking through the rearview mirror of your life, recalling and reclaiming experiences that have shaped your life. It can be a form of an oral or a written history that can bring closure and healing and can serve as a remembrance to younger generations. Several techniques are available to assist in this process, through the use of expressive artwork and the *Living and Leaving A Strengths-Based Legacy* techniques found in this book's Appendix.

Life repair essentially leads us through various stages of the forgiveness process, something almost all of us need to practice. Each day, newspapers and newscasts report events of brutality. They surface in many forms: physical, emotional, social, sexual, political, financial, vocational, and even religious abuse. Though we may deny it, rarely in our society can we come across a person who has not been traumatized in one way or another.

Like physical healing, forgiveness is a process. In their book, *Forgiveness: How to Make Peace With Your Past and Get On With Life*, Sidney and Suzanne Simon list five stages involved in the process (Simon & Simon 1991). They also offer a host of strategies to successfully move through the stages to a time of hope and healing.

One of the specific life repair exercises from Reb Zalman's work that Julia uses during her workshops is called *A Testimonial Dinner for the Severe Teachers* (Schachter-Shalomi 1995). You imagine that those people who have severely hurt you are invited to a dinner. Through imaging or journaling, you invite these people to this celebration. You make a list of the hurt that was done to you, and then list the blessings or lessons learned from that difficult situation. At the end, you picture shaking hands with these people as they leave the celebration. Exercises like this underscore the important message that forgiveness is not about forgetting or condoning, but about removing the residual power of a negative or harmful experience.

The second part of spiritual eldering involves how to age holistically and proactively, harvesting the wisdom of your life and transforming it into a legacy. "It entails discovering the passion and the mystery of the unlived life," Julia informs us. "I've been reading one of Wayne Dyer's books and was struck by the statement, 'Don't die with the music still in you' [Dyer 2002]. For example, many musicians claim to hear music in their heads before it is written on paper or played with an instrument. Another way to say it is that we were all born for a reason, but if we fail to pursue this life purpose, the music of our lives remains unexpressed.

"Speaking personally, I didn't know about my artistic talents until I began to explore my own sense of purpose. It was like someone who always wanted to be a farmer but became a stockbroker instead and later began to explore gardening, finding great joy in it. So it becomes a matter of not following your bliss, of not taking risks, or of being paralyzed by parental and cultural shoulds and oughts."

Sinclair Lewis's Babbitt serves as a poignant example: *"Dad, I can't stand it any more. Maybe [college is] . . . all right for some fellows. But, me, I want to get into mechanics."* Babbitt replies, *"Well . . . now, for heaven's sake, don't repeat this to your mother . . . but practically, I've never done a single thing I've wanted to in my whole life"* (Lewis 1922).

On the other hand, people living in their sixties, and especially baby boomers who are approaching this age, find themselves unusually blessed with many more healthy and productive years. These bonus years offer an opportunity to pursue a new direction; in five years we can be trained to do many things. In addition, the Internet and the knowledge explosion make the possibility of pursuing a life/work passion almost limitless. This can be a time of life to pursue meaning, as opposed to the cultural norm of attempting to stay as young as possible and deny the aging process.

A Day in the Life of an Ideal Elder is one of Julia's exercises from Reb Zalman's work that assists elders to more clearly identify and follow their bliss. This imagery exercise invites a person to determine on a daily basis what she/he would do that brings joy. If a spouse or significant other is involved in one's life, it becomes especially important to share this information and resolve any conflicts.

Julia emphasizes, "Reb Zalman asserts that part of this whole process of being proactive about aging is to make peace with the reality that we will all die and to prepare for this by taking care of the business of making a will and so on. People need to be prepared financially, emotionally, and spiritually, and when this business is taken care of, we can get on with our lives."

Julia utilizes a variety of expressive arts techniques to help people convey their particular story. In her workshop called *My Life as a Work of Art,* she facilitates a process that evolves from the creation of a collage artfully conveying a person's life purpose and legacy. In a period of about three hours, participants cut images and phrases from magazines, forming them into a visual representation of what William Tyndale called the "message wherefore I am sent into the world." She relates, "I am integrating expressive arts into many of my work activities and now work with hospice patients as an expressive arts facilitator. We even do collage work at the bedside.

"I utilize a variety of approaches and adaptations. One involves showing a client a collage tray containing found objectives such as stones, feathers, and other interesting pieces that I have collected. The client then selects the desired items and places them on a mat board where they are glued. People report and interpret what they see. In fact, the 2004 calendar of the Florida hospice where I work includes photos of these collages. Some people are intimidated at the prospect of engaging in traditional art forms, but they resonate with this approach because it is new to them and there is no way to fail. Patients who are unable to pick up objects from the collage tray can give verbal instructions. Even people with dementia can participate in collage-making from magazines. The goal is always the process and not necessarily the outcome."

Julia also works with nurses to create a healing tapestry, a collage expressing their personal healing journey. The contemplative process helps nurses to more consciously depict their professional legacy. Reb Zalman likens this process to reformatting one's hard drive to preserve important data. Nurses might use the information they learned about themselves from processing their art for mentoring other nurses and in communicating strengths and interests during employment interviews or performance discussions.

Touch drawing serves as another one of Julia's art tools (www.touchdrawing.com). It entails a simple process where the fingers take the place of pen or brush. Tissue is placed over a freshly painted board and with fingers, thumbs, or nails, one touches the tissue and makes images, after which the tissue is pulled up and the painting is revealed on the reverse side. The images then become talking points in relating someone's history and current emotional state. Again, it is all about the process of making a creative and caring connection.

Julia reports that some hospice patients use artwork in the form of watercolors to create their personal greeting cards, which then are used to write and send a personal note to someone as a way of saying good-bye and achieving closure. The cards offer people the opportunity to express joy and to make connections. "We view our hospice patients' expressive artwork as an end-of-life legacy left for family," Julia explains.

Julia also recommends that service providers working with elders with dementia consider being trained in *Time Slips,* another expressive arts technique (www.timeslips.com). It is a process whereby a group of people gathers in a circle and creates stories in response to a picture provided by a facilitator. The facilitator copies a picture and distributes it to all participants, asking them to respond with a story line. The leader captures these responses on a large sketchpad, occasionally reading the story back in order to renew the group's focus and energy. At the hour's end, the group is left with a sense of joy and accomplishment. Caregivers who utilize this technique with Alzheimer's patients often report increased alertness and responsiveness.

Stringing beads is another technique Julia uses in helping clients relate their life's journey. "Beads have been used during prayer and meditation for more than 2,000 years, not just in the form of a rosary," she reports. "They are used in almost all faith traditions, so I put beads in a wonderful bowl and allow people to choose which beads they like and then to string them, usually with a piece of elastic. An artist mentor who works with me maintains that often each bead represents some aspect of that person. The other day I worked with a man who was 60 years old, but who was a 4-year-old developmentally. His mother was in her eighties and had been his caregiver his entire life. The man made a necklace for his mother, and it may be the only thing she will ever have as a gift of remembrance from her son."

There is a common thread of communication and sacred connection with others that is woven through all of Julia's work. As an entrepreneur, inspirational teacher, and speaker, she thrives at pushing the creative limits. If you would like additional information about her services, visit her Web site at www.constantsource.com or e-mail her at Julia@constantsource.com.

MONTGOMERY HOSPICE

Beverly Paukstis, RN, MS, CHPN, and Drew Lermond, RN

"One of the reasons many people view hospice as being on the cutting edge of health care is that care is not limited to just the patient," states Beverly Paukstis, Vice President of Clinical Services for Montgomery Hospice in Rockville, Maryland, a suburb of Washington, DC. "The patient and the family together receive services," she explains. "If the family experiences a bad day, it will impact the patient, so both receive care from us. In addition, pain brings with it many components including physical, emotional, financial, and spiritual elements. The other dimensions can heighten the experience of physical pain; therefore, hospice brings a multidisciplinary team to deal with all issues affecting a terminally ill patient."

Beverly and her team enter each person's situation and environment as a guest, asking permission for everything that they do. The patient and the family participate in all of the decisions to be made, even if it involves pain management. To support this approach, every hospice agency must bring its team together at least once every other week to discuss their patients. "We discuss various interventions and document the desired outcome," she states. "Then we work together during the following two weeks to make sure it happens. This tactic is already having an impact on medicine in general."

A United Way agency, Montgomery Hospice has a 25-year heritage and produced one of the first videos on hospice care. Beverly directs both inpatient and home care activities for the agency, which has an average total census of about 140 patients. "We are very fortunate, because our organization is well respected and receives a lot of support from the community," Beverly informs us.

Beverly believes that the ideal time for a person diagnosed with a terminal condition to enter a hospice program is about six months prior to their anticipated death, or at least long enough to work through all of the physical and psycho/social/spiritual issues. "For hospice to break even financially, about 50 days of care is needed because of the initial investment of getting all of the medical equipment in place and meeting intensely with the individual. We like to back off a bit in the middle of the process and then spend more time at the end," Beverly explains. "The final end-of-life work becomes much easier when we are able to establish an intense relationship in the beginning. Unfortunately, we have an average length of stay of about 44 days, which is not unusual nationwide. This represents another unfortunate example of our being a death-denying society."

Like most hospices, Montgomery involves some of its staff members as outreach educators. Much like a detail person for a pharmaceutical company, they visit periodically with physicians, nursing homes, and their staffs. Often they do such things as providing bereavement counseling for office staff when long-term patient relationships terminate.

Beverly believes that one of the hallmarks setting hospice apart from other organizations involves the mandate under the Medicare hospice benefit provision that 5% of patient care hours must be given by volunteers. "The reason for this is varied," she reports. "Most importantly, when volunteers visit a client, they have no agenda. A dying person knows that a nurse continues to return no matter how awful they look or smell and gets a paycheck. But a volunteer who continues to visit is kind in a variety of ways and continues to honor them as a person—that is awesome!"

Volunteers receive training in how to initiate a life review process. Some of them produce videos of patients so their legacies can be preserved. Many hospices also teach volunteers how to do lavender oil hand massage to help relieve anxiety, and some of the larger agencies provide a variety of other integrative therapies such as music, art, and meditation.

Beverly envisions herself continuing to work in hospice or in a similar profession in the future. "It's something you either love or hate. If a person doesn't enjoy this kind of work, she or he won't last very long," she underscores.

Drew Lermond, a hospice nurse, concurs. He especially enjoys getting to know people personally and hearing their life stories. "I love hearing about people's lives," he says. "I had a patient who had been a Marine and witnessed the famous raising of the flag on Iwo Jima.

"Hospice work is difficult but also quite fulfilling," he states. Drew thoroughly enjoys wearing different hats as he relates to patients, not only as nurse, but sometimes almost filling the role of social worker and chaplain. However, he allows the patient and the family to determine much of the conversation and engages in a lot of listening. "You really have to be observant of the patient's non-verbal cues and take some direction from them."

In a new role as the admitting nurse, he explains that he gets the ball rolling for every new patient. "I see every new patient and visit with their families, explaining our services."

A number of the hospice nurses we interviewed for our third book, *The Soul of the Caring Nurse* (Henry & Henry 2004), reported that many people die with a sense of peace and even joy. Drew has also experienced the same phenomenon. "Yes, I have witnessed it in my practice," he reports. "Quite a few of our patients reach a state of acceptance. Of course, some patients lapse into a state of unconsciousness, while others remain coherent up until the time of death and linger in denial. Obviously, we strive for acceptance, but we've had patients fight it until the last heartbeat. One woman I can remember had the most serene look on her face that I have ever seen, and I've served more than 2,000 patients to date. I came home and told my wife that I had just seen the most beautiful dead person. Prior to her passing she had a high degree of near-death awareness, hearing music and other good things."

Drew believes that how a person lives during a lifetime impacts how they approach death. "I think it has more to do with how someone has lived their life rather than age that makes the difference," he believes. "Some children often seem to hold on to life, whereas those who believe that they have achieved their sense of purpose in life are more apt to pass over."

Drew frequently uses the words "passed on" or "passed over" when talking about patients. Asked if his use of language was intentional, he explains.,"Yes; I am a Christian, but I honor all faith systems. However you describe your faith, passing over is a process. I have enjoyed being able to witness patients in this respect and have read books like *Final Gifts* [Callahan & Kelley 1992]. But, who is to say what form it takes?"

Drew calls upon his intuition in terms of when it is appropriate to discuss end-of-life issues with a patient and their family. "Some people don't even want to hear the word 'hospice,' while others express openly the belief that they are dying." He believes that it is necessary to be honest about the diagnosis, but in a tactful and compassionate manner. A small percentage of the people who enter hospice experience an improvement in their health and eventually leave the program. "I explain to them in terms of the guy upstairs telling us when to get on the bus," he affirms. "We've experienced patients who have made a remarkable turnaround. I tell people that their fate is not written in stone. Also, hospice may not be about curing, but it doesn't mean we are not going to care for you. We will be caring for you differently, perhaps even better, because our approach is holistic. People who have received a terminal diagnosis have an opportunity, if they choose, to gain new knowledge and to pass it on as part of a legacy.

"Even when someone becomes quite lethargic and tends to sleep most of the time, I will tell the family that Mom or Dad may not respond cognitively, but it doesn't mean that they can't hear you. Therefore, they may say whatever is in the heart."

Hearing Drew and other workers speak about hospice, we can't help concluding that they are therapists in the broadest sense of the word. They not only deal with the physical symptoms of an illness and help to manage pain, but in many different ways they serve as channels for healing energy.

Adopting an Elder

Amy Brown, BSN, RN

When Boulder, Colorado, psychiatric nurse Amy Brown and her partner "adopted" a dear friend who had been diagnosed with early dementia about nine years ago, her passion for eldercare was extended beyond her professional nursing work. As a hospital case manager, she works largely with elders and their families who need to problem solve and develop care strategies. "Obviously, most people want to remain independent in their own home," she says, "but a hospital visit often becomes the first time that desire is challenged. Because of Medicare requirements, many patients are discharged to a rehabilitation facility for a period of time, giving them a snapshot of what that is like. Unlike what they may believe, a short-term stay in a nursing home is not always the end of living independently. We do a lot of 'layering,' using the hospital and rehab to get as many services as possible, and then to increase or decrease them as necessary after recovery. While people really want to remain at home, I see the need for more creative alternatives such at the Eden Alternative™-type developments and community housing projects, which support aging in place.

"How to age well and creatively is a very timely concern," Amy recounts. "Somehow we need to manage the aging process and visualize how to do it differently than today's norm. I hear a well-intentioned concern about this subject across many disciplines." Adopting her elder friend is one creative example of eldercaring.

"Marilyn was a single, retired school teacher living independently, but with very limited family and relative connections. We became more socially involved with her, but then noticed changes, especially when she was no longer able to drive her car," Amy reports. "Over time, we witnessed significant changes in her self-care and level of independent functioning. We slowly became more involved in her life and she knew that she had someone to reply upon, helping with some of the household chores and taking her to doctor's appointments.

"This continued for about 30 months until we became more concerned about safety issues. It was a sad story in the sense that her loss of family of origin left her as a kind of orphan. In fact, many 'orphan elders' exist in our society. We need a more

163

formal elder adoption system in this country because, like children, many of them need families and support."

A small number of such programs apparently exist in the United States. For example, in principle, the Adopt an Elder Foundation in California believes that every person and their family deserve the right to choose how they age and how the delivery of care will be administered (www.adoptanelder.org). Designed to subsidize low-income, Medi-Cal-eligible seniors needing daily care and supervision in an assisted living community, this program saves thousands of dollars monthly by preventing premature placement in a nursing home.

In addition, gerontologist John Gibson (mentioned earlier) and co-author Judy Pigott envision a "sharing the care" movement taking place in this country in response to baby boomers, along with other groups in need, facing overwhelming eldercare demands and unplanned and/or unwelcome changes in their own lives. Their upcoming book will include chapters on asking for help, when a care team is needed, how it is formed, and how to keep it going. Volunteer teams could be formed and coordinated by community resource centers, faith-related communities, and health clinics, as well as any organization with a community-oriented service initiative.

Fortunately for Amy and her partner, Marilyn was quite open to their increasing support. She spoke quite often about having Alzheimer's. Slowly, therefore, it became possible for them to increase visits and participate in her life. Then, three years ago she sold her condo, and the three of them purchased a home with enough room for an apartment for Marilyn. "She especially needed the socialization and the availability of 24-hour support; thus we became a blended family," Amy relates. "We were very lucky in that we were able to hire a seasoned caregiver to serve as a companion during the daytime while my partner and I were at work. Marilyn spent the majority of her time enjoying our yard and spent some spiritual solitude surrounded by her cat and our dogs."

For others who may be providing home care for a person with Alzheimer's, Amy highly recommends a book by Mary Summer Rain entitled *Love Never Sleeps: Living at Home With Alzheimer's* (Rain 2002). It is clearly written so lay people can understand it, yet packed with insights for the professional as well.

By providing this space along with personal, loving care, Amy and her partner were able to create an environment conducive to flowering the seeds of gero-transcendence. Marilyn experienced quality, intimate companionship, a connection with her beloved nature and animals, as well as positive solitude so important to the nurturing of an elder's soul. "She could sit for hours and pet the dogs in a kind of meditative, satisfying simplicity," Amy affirms. "All of the things they tell you to do during early and middle stages of Alzheimer's were at her fingertips—touch, music, nature, animals, and the like." At least in part, this allows for a natural progression toward maturation, even when the person is afflicted with a disease of some kind.

The environment Amy and her partner created for Marilyn was somewhat akin to the Windhorse model. Developed in the 1980s by Dr. Edward Podvoll and his colleagues at Naropa University in Boulder, its focus is upon treating various mental problems including those associated with aging. Windhorse was a mythic horse symbolizing a person's energy and discipline to uplift him/her. In this model, the core approach involves surrounding a person with enough structure and sanity to positively impact their dysfunctional situation. It entails keeping a person out of an institution and into a therapeutic home and community setting. People's lives can be stabilized not only through pharmacology but also because of caring, loving interpersonal relationships.

After about 2-1/2 years, Marilyn experienced a fairly radical downward change in her Alzheimer's disease and in her physical health. Interestingly, Marilyn herself began speaking about going to a facility, according to Amy. So in the fall of 2004 they moved her to a small home serving only six residents that embraced a very therapeutic family-oriented model. Staff members and students from Naropa University worked with a holistic approach using aromatherapy, massage, and music, utilizing several of the senses. "Unfortunately," Amy sadly recounts, "the facility had to close its doors, symptomatic of how independent services seem to be struggling financially these days. We moved Marilyn into a new, larger, and memory-impairment-focused environment. Living with her taught me firsthand how important the environment is, especially with people suffering from dementia and Alzheimer's. It needs to be calm and soothing as well as structured. Memory-impaired individuals need a balance to keep them engaged and stimulated and to allow time for quietness and reflection."

Amy confirmed for us that living in a holistic-oriented, caring environment makes a significant difference. "During her earlier years, Marilyn lived alone and hospitalized herself several times because of panic and anxiety attacks. When she moved in with us and entered a reliable, caring setting, they ceased and she never again called 911. Even today as she moves into the advanced stages of Alzheimer's, she exhibits a kind of other-directedness, asking 'How are you doing?' This is amazing to me when you consider that someone's mind is changing."

Considering her nursing work of caring for patients on a daily basis, we asked Amy why in the world she would want to adopt an elder, especially one with dementia. "Quite honestly," she replied, "it is really about what I can learn and about keeping alive the essence and spirit of another person. It's about a basic human gift that we can give to one another, a responsibility to take care of each other. It's like coming home and having your kids take you back to what is most important. Marilyn would pull me out of the busyness of the day as we would simply go for a purposeless walk or have a good meal together and share in laughter."

Again, we have an excellent testimony to what elders are good for in terms of the attributes of "being." They can teach us the values of receptivity, basic life and human worth, simplicity, and child-like innocence.

Even though today Marilyn resides in an assisted living facility, Amy and her partner visit her on a regular basis. Caring for her is no longer a marathon as it was when they lived together. "But," she asserts after some reflection, "I would do it again because I believe that all elderly people are vitally important. It is the right thing to do. They are human beings with essence and deserve our respect and gratitude. Even with her disease, Marilyn has spirit and real meaning, threads of which come through even in the most difficult of circumstances; that is what we are spending our time with."

MUSIC HEALING PRACTITIONER

Kathleen Masters, RN, BSN

Several years ago Jim heard Harvard-trained theoretical physicist Dr. John Hagelin address a conference on science and spirituality. He went to the blackboard and for 20 minutes worked his way through mathematical equations, none of which were understood. Finally, he turned around and said, "Now what this means is that God is music."

Someone else at the conference mentioned the composer Sergei Rachmaninoff who responded, when asked how he came to write his music, "I go into a room by myself, sit down, and listen to the music. When it stops, I write it down."

Kathleen Masters, RN, BSN, a music healing practitioner, affirms this perception. "I believe that the universe is connected by vibrations that can affect us both positively and negatively at the cellular level," she states. Based upon prevailing views of quantum physicists, in our book, *Reclaiming Soul in Health Care*, we describe the universe as being essentially living, organic energy, a harmonious invisible whole (Henry & Henry 1999). Kathleen uses the word *vibration*. "We know that we are vibratory beings," she affirms. "This is why sound affects us on a cellular level and why we get a response from the resonance.

"According to Joshua Leeds, sound researcher and composer, in his book, *The Power of Sound* [Leeds 2001], resonance is 'the frequency at which an object most naturally vibrates,'" explains Kathleen. "Leeds goes on to broaden the definition to include, 'the impact of one vibration on another.' We are affected by every sound with which we come into contact. Most of us can recall the sounds of construction on a busy street. The pounding jackhammers and rumbling trucks send out vibrations that disturb our cells' natural vibration. We want to leave the noise behind and find some calmness. So, we seek resonance by turning our car radios to the classical station or putting on a favorite CD. Our cells are soothed by the cello or soft piano music and regain some measure of balance. Music practitioners intentionally choose sound/music to create a particular resonance with a patient/client."

The recognition of the importance of music and sound is not new. Based on the belief that every sickness is a musical problem and every answer is musical, music has been used by shamans for over 5000 years. John Armstrong, in his *Art of Preserving Health,* extols the virtue of music: "Music exalts each Joy, allays each Grief, expels Diseases, softens every Pain, subdues the rage of Poison and the Plague" (Armstrong 1744, I, p. 512). Pat Moffitt Cook, Director of Open Ear Center, Bainbridge Island, Washington, uses musical remedies to "stimulate physical and emotional balance, releasing stagnating energy and reconnecting people with a dynamic stillness within." According to Kathleen, the human body matches its rhythms to the sounds of the music being played, which is called entrainment. Thus, by presenting more soothing and relaxing sounds, it is possible to help people move to a more calming place.

Kathleen describes how the use of music and sound within clinical settings can facilitate one's self-healing capacities and is demonstrated to be useful in reducing stress and anxiety, pain, and the nausea and vomiting associated with chemotherapy. Among other areas where music has been found effective to reduce symptoms or improve recovery include brain damage following head trauma, dementia, hypertension and cardiac arrhythmia, and with Parkinson's disease and in stroke recovery. Music is useful in calming patients with Alzheimer's disease, since music memory is embedded in a different part of the brain. And, the use of music aids in the transition process of dying. "Different instruments can help people move out of their bodies," she explains.

The use of music is increasingly being used within operating rooms to aid in the relaxation of patients receiving anesthesia who may then require less medication and often heal faster. "I have a set of recordings that may be listened to before entering surgery and even while under anesthesia. The combination of spoken affirmations for healing with soothing music recorded to synchronize both brain hemispheres encourages the patient's body, mind, and spirit toward healing," Kathleen notes.

Kathleen's personal journey toward transformational change began by reconnecting to music. "I was raised in a musical family," Kathleen affirms. "My three brothers and I always sang in school and church choirs. Then, in 1995 a nurse friend of mine gave me some reference material about using music at the bedside. One of the books happened to be the *The Mozart Effect,* by Don Campbell (Campbell 2001). Later, I attended one of his four-weekend conferences on the transforming effect of sound that stirred my spirit to explore this potent medium that has stimulated and accompanied mankind's search for health in all its forms through the ages.

"Pat Moffit Cook's workshops are geared toward health practitioners on how to use cross-cultural, recorded music at the bedside or during a therapeutic session. She incorporates sounds from other cultures, both chanted and played on musical instruments, because they have certain acoustical elements in them. For instance, a drone, such as the Australian digeridoo or guttural chanting of Tibetan monks, has a grounding effect. The use of high-frequency sounds seems to awaken the mind or distract the patient away from pain. My three-year work with Dr. Cook has broadened and expanded my world of practical resources to use with patients as well as myself." Kathleen also recommends *Biomedical Foundations of Music as Therapy* as an additional reference (Taylor 1997). "Dr. Dale Taylor speaks about the use of music specifically for conditions like strokes, Parkinson's disease, and dementia. The receptors for music are located in a different part of the brain, allowing people to enjoy the experience of hearing the music."

Another book that is dear to her is *The World is Sound*, written by Joachim-Ernst Berendt, a foremost European jazz producer who explored musical traditions in diverse cultures and who reaffirms what ancient people have always known—the world is sound, rhythm, and vibration (Berendt 1983).

Also trained in Therapeutic Touch, Kathleen has used the approach as an adjunct to nursing as an energetic, non-invasive way to help calm people and reduce pain. Developed by two women the 1970s, Therapeutic Touch methodology involves a process of energy direction and modulation using the hands to facilitate and encourage healing. A scientifically based practice developed by Dolores Krieger, PhD, RN, formerly a Professor at New York University, and Dora Kunz, gifted healer and past President of the Theosophical Society, it views the human energy field as governed by pattern and order. "For me, it also involves a way to send compassionate feeling from me to a patient," Kathleen underscores. "My intention is to send them the message that someone has slowed down enough to be fully present in their lives, listening to what they need at that precise moment."

Kathleen currently works as a home health and hospice nurse and previously worked in an emergency department. Kathleen utilizes music and sound in her workshops and, because she is fairly new in her current job, she has yet to introduce it to her clients, although she hopes to add this dimension to her nursing care in the future. "At the moment," she relates, "my practice is grounded in being present from my heart with my patients. In every visit, I practice 'presence,' centering myself so that I am totally connecting with them as the spirit leads. We have some extraordinary experiences, entering into what is called 'timeless time.' If a person is completely present, linear, chronological time dissipates into 'kairos,' a Greek word used to describe quality 'I-Thou' moments. At such a time, the patient *knows* that you are there for them, even while performing a clinical procedure. It appears as though we invested a half hour of service and received three times as much from it. Time seems to expand as I sit with a patient and perhaps a family member and completely give myself to that moment."

We asked Kathleen to respond to a hypothetical situation where one of us received a terminal diagnosis of living for no more than six months. Could she work with us in setting up music therapy regimentation? "Absolutely!" she says emphatically. "I would conduct an intake interview, finding out your likes and dislikes with respect to music. Beyond this, perhaps we would explore issues that you would like to put to rest before you died. Music would be used to help you through the process of letting go of them. We might apply the issues to the seven chakras and use music specifically composed for them. For example, there is heart chakra music, and I used it with a cardiac patient who had a very rapid heartbeat and experienced anxiety attacks.

Through the music, she was able to identify the grief causing the cardiac problems and anxiety. She subsequently gained some confidence and began to practice meditation."

In her private practice, Kathleen uses music as part of the diagnostic process. "The client listens to music and then reports what feelings and thoughts are brought to the surface. It is similar to journaling about a dream. Music can carry us to deeper places, bringing body, mind, and spirit together."

Music can have a positive effect upon caregivers as well as care receivers. Elder caregivers in particular find the caregiving process quite stressful. For this reason, Kathleen offers a workshop entitled *Music for Self Health*. She speaks about the use of toning, chanting, and humming for personal benefit. "I would love to see this practice expanded for caregivers," she states. "I've also thought of instituting music respite breaks in clinical settings. I conducted a study of such five-minute breaks during my work in the emergency department. It made an incredible difference as my ER colleagues experienced an oasis of calm music. Because of the trickle-down effect, this may be more important for the caregivers than for the patients or clients. Imagine a healthcare setting where the practitioners are able to use tools such as humming and toning, as well as listening to soothing music, to keep them[selves] healthy."

As she drives from one client to another, Kathleen listens to a wide variety of music. One of her favorites is the very soothing instrumental music of Brian Crain. Examples of his music can be accessed at www.briancrain.com. "I am also very drawn to flute music, such as that of Tibetan musician Nawang Khechog or Native American Carlos Nakai."

In her practice, Kathleen works with a large number of elders with varying stages of dementia. "It is absolutely true that while these people may be declining in terms of cognitive abilities, their spirit remains intact. People with dementia, as well as those at the end of life, tend to discard their personas or masks. The filters or impulse controls they impose upon themselves disappear, so they become more childlike and open. They don't have an agenda, which in many ways represents a gift as compared to a 40-year-old person in the emergency room with chest pains. I find them living in a very simplified way that allows for extraordinary communication."

As such, Kathleen affirms the statement in scripture, "Whoever does not receive the kingdom of God like a child shall not enter it" (Mark 10:15 RSV). She believes this holds true at many levels. This statement probably refers to the primary energy of "being" discussed in Section 1. Bill Thomas speaks about our current obsession with the "doing" dimensions, with activity, performance, and making our mark in the world. As people move into elderhood, this obsession loses some of its power and, in holistic aging, "being" surfaces in significance. This is very much the experience of Kathleen as she works with her more elderly clients. "My sense is sometimes their response represents a mild form of surprise that someone wants to be present with them," she responds.

Both children and holistic-oriented elders tend to display receptive, open-minded behaviors more conducive to cosmic energies. "It reflects an open heart that children have not learned to cover up yet and which I experience with many elders," Kathleen quietly acknowledges. "Especially with dementia, perhaps not by choice, but the impulse to cover up seems to disappear. I know that some people with dementia are very angry and paranoid, but I'm speaking of people like my aunt who, when I visit her, always seems to be singing a song."

A growing number of elders live at home well into their eighties and nineties without any need for home health care. Kathleen dreams of serving as a consultant to such people. "Not associated with a particular organization, I would function as a holistic nurse utilizing a number of modalities. From my perspective, there are many inexpensive and portable practices we could offer to clients and their families."

When asked to describe her current sense of life legacy, she replies, "I believe I am called to bring compassionate presence into the practice of nursing and to health care as a whole. I truly feel that today I serve as a role model in this respect."

THE HEALING POWER OF TRUST

Liz Hopkins, RN, C

Liz Hopkins credits the "Holistic Health" and "Dying and Death" university classes she took during the course of obtaining her BSN degree with expanding her insight into the role that *trust* plays between a caregiver and a patient or client. She currently works as the clinical manager of the medical renal unit at St. Peter's Hospital in Olympia, Washington. She has geriatric certification, and her experience includes 16 years working in a nursing home.

"I absolutely loved our Holistic Health professor, Jane Cornman, PhD, RN," she states enthusiastically, "because she was so passionate about the subject. I learned how different people process their healing and interact with their healers. In virtually all instances, the matter of trust was the important factor in the interaction between the caregiver and the patient or client. The higher the degree of trust, the higher the possibility became of a positive outcome. The course opened my mind to the many holistic options available. I particularly found the Tibetan 'singing bowl' intriguing, which I learned can be a very effective resource for healing when used with someone who has trust and faith in the process."

The existence of singing bowls dates back to a period of the historical Buddha Shakyamunie (560–480 BC). Along with the teachings of Buddha, the bowls were brought to Tibet from India. Traditionally constructed of a seven-metal alloy, said to include gold, silver, copper, iron, lead, tin, and mercury, the bowls are most often used as meditation aids and can be found on private Buddhist altars and in temples, monasteries, and meditation halls around the world. The sounds of the bowls have been found to be relaxing and soothing. In addition to their use in meditation, the bowls are used for deep relaxation, stress reduction, holistic healing, Reiki, chakra balancing, and world music.

"People with kidney failure are very sick," Liz relates, "and experience the failure of multiple systems. Anything that can bring them comfort other than just medication represents a wonderful opportunity. Again, the trust factor becomes a necessary component of any effective method of healing. Personally, I love the laying on of hands and believe in Healing Touch."

Liz enjoys using a number of therapies in caring for herself. "On my day off, one of the first things I do is to light candles and enjoy their aroma. I pick scents that provide me with comfort. Unfortunately, the hospital setting is not very conducive to using aromas. However, they could be effectively used in nursing homes to mask some of the institutional smells."

Liz claims that the class she attended on dying and death represented one of the best educational experiences she has had. Information included learning about the experiences of dying within different cultures. "During the last three years, I lost both my father and mother-in-law," she reports, "so the course was quite relevant. We learned about how people live with the thought of dying, about how people change and interact with their families during the process, and about expectations after death. The emphasis was upon treating people with respect and allowing them to come to whatever closure was necessary.

"Working in a nursing home, I came in contact with many, many dying experiences. People need to get their mental and emotional affairs in order. For example, my Dad felt an urgent need to tell us about his experiences as a child. He wanted to preserve these stories through his children. It doesn't matter about the nature of the need; the caregiver must be sensitive to it and allow people their choices."

Regardless of its nature, Liz believes that people with a strong faith system tend to experience less fear and anxiety as they pass through the end stages of life. As the body begins to close down, they enjoy the presence and prayers of others in their faith tradition. The atmosphere could be described as being more calm and peaceful. The notion that when we die we are going someplace else especially brings some solace. "However," she underscores, "it remains important to understand that everyone is an individual and may have diverse beliefs and experiences. It becomes very important to have a kind of 'point person' who seeks out what is wanted and works to make it happen if possible."

In one form or another, in reality, this kind of education is vitally important for everyone, especially in a culture which is largely in death denial. "Contrast this with a terminally ill native American Indian patient in our unit last week. For almost a week, 30 or more relatives kept rotating through her room in a very quiet and accepting manner, knowing that death was close by. It was quite unusual compared with other situations where no one acknowledges the dying process. The cultural difference was heartwarming."

Not surprising, Liz has prepared for her own eventual death, and not just in terms of making a will. She and her family will find comfort in their Catholic faith. She also prepares through setting a good example, living the values that she professes are dear to her. "I even have my obituary written, which was part of the class I took on dying and death," she relates.

AGING AND HIV/AIDS

Charles A. Emlet, PhD, ACSW

"At the time I began HIV work in the 1980s, life expectancy after an AIDS diagnosis was somewhere between 6 and 24 months," explains Dr. Charles Emlet, Associate Professor of Social Work at the University of Washington, Tacoma. "To be older with AIDS at that time, one had to be diagnosed in late life. There are now two distinct populations of older adults with HIV/AIDS: those diagnosed later in life and those long-term survivors who can now grow old with this disease."

Because of its serious nature and the stigma often associated with it, eldercare providers need to have some insight into the relationship of aging and HIV. HIV is a virus that damages the immune system. HIV infection leads to a much more serious disease called AIDS. When HIV infects the body, the immune system can weaken. This puts a person in danger of getting other life-threatening diseases, infections, and cancers. When that happens, AIDS occurs, the last stage of HIV infection.

Nationally recognized for his work in this arena and the editor of a book on the subject of aging and HIV/AIDS, Dr. Emlet has conducted research which has taken a variety of shapes and approaches (Emlet 2004). It has included secondary analysis of existing data, a two-year quantitative study, and a mixed-methods study that includes the gathering of quantitative data along with qualitative interviews. He informs us, "If we are going to understand HIV/AIDS among older people, we need to see it in its historical context. AIDS in an older individual was first documented as a case study in 1986 when a 57-year-old man, diagnosed with Alzheimer's disease, was found on autopsy to have progressive dementia caused by HTLV-III (the term used at that time for HIV)" (Emlet 2005).

In terms of demographics, the data from national, state, and local sources suggests a slow but consistent "graying" of HIV in this country. During a period from 1994 to 2000, the median age at diagnosis with AIDS in the U.S. has risen from 37 to 39 years.

"If we are going to make progress in areas of education and prevention, one of the issues we need to confront is the attitudes and beliefs of the public, older adults as well as medical and service providers, about aging and sexuality. Such misconception and ageist attitudes surrounding aging and sexuality are infused in our society, resulting in poor prevention efforts, unnecessary infections, delayed diagnosis, misdiagnosis, and ultimately unnecessary deaths. Despite the fact that AIDS among older persons was first acknowledged nearly 20 years ago, misconceptions continue. Older people are seen as asexual, and if by some strange chance they manage to have sex, they are [believed to be] obviously heterosexual and certainly monogamous. Additionally, our inability to acknowledge older persons' use of illicit drugs seems systemic" (Emlet 2005).

> *"The younger ones can't change as fast. I mean if my roommate was to throw me out tomorrow, fine. I'll go find someplace else to live. I'm not as scared, I've started over before, and I'll do it again if I have to."*
> —Pete, age 51
>
> *"It's [age] majestic. Half a century. Right there with Mt. Rainier."*
> —Ellie, age 59

HIV is a disease transmitted through unprotected sex and exposure to contaminated blood. Older adults, despite our strong denial, are exposed to HIV by the same means as younger persons. These risk factors will certainly continue to increase in the coming years with the aging of the baby boom generation and their generational mindset related to drug use and sexuality.

An important element that affects the quality of life of all persons with HIV disease is stigma. "Even though we have entered the third decade of the pandemic, HIV stigma continues to exist and is therefore deserving of study," Dr. Emlet believes. "Stigma associated with HIV has been defined as prejudice, discounting, discrediting, and discrimination directed at people perceived to have HIV or AIDS." According to Bergen and colleagues and illustrated below, stigma can be described in three subsets (Bergen, Ferrans, & Lashley 2001). *Personalized stigma* is associated with such factors as feelings of isolation and rejection as well as experiences of negative rela-

> *"I just think that people who are living with HIV over 50 have a huge responsibility to be educators. My position has always been that I'm more concerned for the next generation than I am for myself."*
>
> —Christa, age 64

tions with others due to HIV. *Negative self-image* includes feelings of guilt, shame, and self-deprecation. *Public attitude* includes social discomfort of being around people with HIV as well as discrimination. Terry (not his real name), who is 51, puts it this way: "The discrimination is a problem for us. A lot of times if you tell somebody, you know, they'll back off and they'll judge you."

Despite the complex physical and social issues faced by many of these individuals, there are consistent themes of survival, resilience, and even generativity, and a concern for others. Dr. Emlet reports, "Pete and Ellie portray a spirit of survivorship, Pete communicating a profound sense of resilience while Ellie compares herself to Mt. Rainier as a survivor."

"Beyond resilience, generativity—a term coined by Erik Erikson—suggests a concern and mentoring responsibility toward others. Several of these older informants discussed a deep need to see beyond their own situation and to reach out to other, younger, individuals" (Emlet 2005).

HIV/AIDS guidelines for eldercare service providers:

▌ Don't assume that older adults are at lesser risk because they are less sexually active. Ask older adults about their sex lives and drug use.
▌ Do anticipate that older people may be less knowledgeable about the disease.
▌ Encourage everyone who has engaged in behaviors associated with HIV risk to get tested for HIV.
▌ Encourage people with HIV to seek out and participate in a support network.
▌ Encourage elders who care for grandchildren to become familiar with the subject of HIV/AIDS.

References

Armstrong, J. 1744. *The Art of Preserving Health.* http://www.giga-usa.com/quotes/authors/john_armstrong_a001.htm (accessed July 30, 2006).

Berendt, J. 1983. *The World is Sound.* Rochester, UT: Destiny Books.

Bergen, B.E., C.E. Ferrans, & F.R. Lashley. 2001. Measuring stigma in people with HIV: Psychometric assessment of the stigma scale. *Research in Nursing and Health* 24: 518–29.

Brand, D. & P. Yancey. 1997. *The Gift of Pain.* Grand Rapids, MI: Zondervan Publishing.

Callahan, M. & P. Kelley. 1992. *Final Gifts.* NY: Bantam Books.

Campbell, D. 2001. *The Mozart Effect.* NY: HarperCollins.

Campbell, J. 1988. *The Power of Myth.* NY: Doubleday.

Clark, B. 1978. *Whose Life Is It?* New York: Avon Books.

Dyer, W. 2002. *Ten Secrets for Success and Inner Peace.* Carlsbad, CA: Hay House.

Emlet, C. 2004. *HIV/AIDS and Older Adults: Challenges for Individuals, Families and Communities.* NY: Springer Publishers.

Emlet, C. 2005. *Aging and HIV/AIDS*: Lessons Learned . . . Moving Forward. Distinguished Research Lecture delivered at the University of Washington, Tacoma. Available at: http://www.tacoma.washington.edu/library/resources/dra.htm (accessed July 30, 2006).

Henry, L. & J. Henry. 1999. *Reclaiming Soul in Health Care.* Chicago: AHA Press.

Henry, L. & J. Henry. 2004. *The Soul of the Caring Nurse.* Silver Springs, MD: Nursesbooks.org., the publishing arm of the ANA.

Kataria, M. 2002. *Laugh for No Reason.* Mumbai, India: Madhuri International.

Leeds, J. 2001. *The Power of Sound.* Rochester, Vermont: Healing Arts Press.

Lewis, S. 1922. *Babbitt.* San Diego: Harcourt Brace Jovanovich.

Piper, W. 1976. *The Little Engine That Could.* NY: Platt and Munk.

Rain, M. 2002. *Love Never Sleeps: Living at Home With Alzheimer's*. Charlottesville, VA: Hampton Roads.

Rantz M., M. Zwygart-Stauffacher, & M. Flesner. 2005. Advances in measuring quality of care in nursing homes: A new tool for providers, consumers, regulators, and researchers. *Journal of Nursing Care Quality*. 20(4):293-6.

Schachter-Shalomi, Z. 1995. *From Age-ing to Sage-ing: A Profound New Vision of Growing Older*. New York: Warner Books.

Simon, S. & S. Simon. 1991. *Forgiveness: How to Make Peace With Your Past and Get On With Life*. New York: Warner Books.

Taylor, D. 1997. *Biomedical Foundations of Music as Therapy*. St. Louis: MMB Music, Inc.

Tornstam, L. 2005. *Gerotranscendence*. New York: Springer Publishing Company.

Wadensten, B. and M. Carlsson. 2002. Theory-driven guidelines for practical care of older people, based on the theory of gerotranscendence. *J Adv Nursing* 36(5):635–42.

Closing Reflections

"Mirror, mirror on the wall, who is fairest of all?," asks Snow White's wicked stepmother in the classic tale, *Snow White and the Seven Dwarfs.* Based upon the testimony of the 37 eldercare professionals whom we interviewed for this book, instead of Snow White or the wicked stepmother, is it possible that the magical, talking mirror might proclaim, "Thou, O *elder*, art the fairest of them all"? While elders may not be the "fairest" in terms of cultural norms for beauty, because of their age and life experiences, they could easily be described as the "fairest" by other standards. Old age offers the possibility of "seeing" more clearly because it connects life's beginnings with its endings. By current research standards, we may see elders as having the *fairest* social, psychological, and spiritual strengths, enabling elders to further develop their talents and contribute to society.

Ageism: A Fundamental Distortion

The first task in "seeing" elders differently entails confronting rampant cultural ageism. As mentioned in Section 1, gerontologist and Pulitzer Prize-winning president of the International Longevity Center-USA, Robert Butler, MD, defines ageism as a "deep seated uneasiness on the part of the young and middle-aged [as well as elders themselves]—a personal revulsion to and distaste for growing old, disease, disability; and fear of

> *"Life and death flow into one, and there is neither evolution nor eternity, only Being."*
> —Albert Einstein

powerlessness, 'uselessness' and death" (Butler 1969). Programmed to view elders in this manner, many of those aged 65 and over look into the mirror and see themselves reflected only as wrinkled relics.

The *Encyclopedia of Ageism* contains over 300 entries. It demonstrates that ageism is perpetuated in many ways, including through advertising, in various art forms, through children, and in politics (Palmore, Branch, & Harris 2005).

Being: A Fundamental Grounding

As mentioned, according to Bill Thomas, MD, an orientation toward *being* is one of the fundamental strengths of many elders (Thomas 2004). *Being,* as opposed to an adult fixation on *doing* and performance, serves as the foundation for understanding elderhood.

Elders are not just older adults any more than children are young adults. Older people bring a wealth of experience and wisdom to the table. They enjoy a tremendous capacity for continued growth.

In his chapter in *Religion, Spirituality, and Aging,* Eugene Bianchi, PhD, reports the results of interviews with more than 100 creative elders (Moody 2005a). Their strengths compare quite favorably with the research of Lars Tornstam on gerotranscendence, introduced earlier, as exemplified in the table below.

The dictate that elders are not just older adults is especially applicable to elder health care. As Sarah Kagan, PhD, RN, gerontological associate professor, University of Pennsylvania School of Nursing, reminds us, "Today, we have a foundational understanding of what it means to age and it needs to be shared with almost all caregivers." As we found, elders' health care needs are different and hospital care can be toxic to this group.

Fortunately, a growing number of elder care providers and age-related organizations are becoming more engaged in transformational eldercare. They are advocating for a change in how we view our elders, exploring new concepts of care and envisioning new models of community, enabling them to "live until they die." During

ELDER STRENGTHS — BIANCHI	ELDER STRENGTHS — TORNSTAM
Heightened self-esteem	Accepting oneself as a unique individual Discovering and accepting hidden aspects of oneself
Harvesting memories	Recalling past experiences
Life-long learning	Calling upon an extensive knowledge system
Expressions of humor	Acting childlike at times but with all the "smarts"
Expressions of gratitude	Appreciating the mystery of life Living simply and rejoicing in simple pleasures
Encountering mortality	Accepting with little or no fear one's mortality
Sense of purpose	Sensing that life has meaning and purpose
Open to possibilities	Openness to new experiences
Fostering more freedom	Withholding judgments and accepting people for what they are Giving unconditional positive regard
Cultivating family and friends	Enjoying quality relationships
Forming intentional communities	Developing and calling upon a strong social system
Fostering peace, justice, and ecology	Promoting cooperation, collaboration, and peace Sensing a kind of oneness with nature

our research, we identified a partial list of more than 50 such organizations. Many professionals engaged in eldercare are baby boomers who have a vested interest in changing attitudes and reforming services. Definitely, the people we interviewed for this book are passionate about their professions.

As we said in the beginning, we do not mean to imply that the emerging concepts and models we highlighted in the stories we included are the only ones that exist. Undoubtedly, there are others that are and will make a transformational difference in eldercare. We simply invite you to consider these, and hopefully they will serve to inspire your own situation, whatever that may be.

Truly, if we are to age well and to live until we die, we must transform our perceptions about aging and eldercare in general. Through the action of one individual, Rosa Parks sparked the modern-day civil rights movement. Those who are quietly going about the work of transforming eldercare are often doing it one organization or one individual at a time. Our wish is that transformational eldercare will become universal—another nationwide movement. Not only is caring for an aging population in ways that are respectful and honoring the *right* thing to do, ultimately, we *do* it for ourselves.

We invite you, our readers, to share your comments and thoughts. We may be reached at jlhenry@aol.com.

Appendix
Living and Leaving a Strengths-Based Legacy: Life Purpose Doesn't End at Age 65 or 95

In his book, *What Are Old People For?* Bill Thomas, MD, introduces the word *senescence* to describe the transitional period between adulthood and elderhood (Thomas 2004). It can be a time of ripening, of reflecting upon one's life experiences, and of capturing periods of richness that help to formulate a sense of one's life purpose and legacy. Typically, the word *legacy* is used to describe a monetary gift given by a donor to an institution or common cause. In fact, the dictionary defines it as *a gift of personal property by will.* However, it can enjoy a much broader perspective. William Tyndale called a legacy the "message wherefore I am sent into the world."

Unfortunately, as mentioned in Section 1, our Western culture tends to view elderhood as a problem to be solved rather than an opportunity to be lived. It is viewed as a time of retirement, leisure, and the gradual diminishment of strengths. As elders age, greater attention is given to deficits and to frailties, erasing prized interests, values, experiences, and non-physical abilities.

Elders often experience financial difficulties, cognitive decline, and loss of family and friends. However, when we focus attention upon a person's strengths, their problems loom less large. Many elders have more time to volunteer, bestowing blessings on others as well as themselves.

We suggest that three themes can be applied to the task of exploring, living, and leaving a strengths-based legacy:

Connecting With Oneself

Connecting with oneself includes entering a life review process. One way to discern your sense of legacy involves looking through an imaginary rearview mirror, recapturing key, passionate life/work events. Over the years, as a career guidance professional having worked with dozens of people in this respect, Jim's experience is that a pattern almost always emerges.

Recount your life story and identify several key, mountaintop experiences. Perhaps a parent, brother, or sister might help you. Or, old scrapbooks may be of assistance to jog your memory. These might be termed moments of *kairos*, a Greek word used to describe prophetic moments and quality events. For our purposes, we are using the word to describe times when you felt engaged and connected by being able to utilize your key, passionate talents and skills. You seem to lose track of time during such a period, an hour appearing to be only ten minutes because you are so occupied. In addition, legacies can spring from negative "pit" experiences, such as for some Mothers Against Drunk Driving (MADD).

A second strategy entails completing inventories such as the Myers-Briggs Type Indicator® (MBTI) that help you to more clearly identify personal strengths. A free version of the MBTI called the Jung Typology Test (not really a test) is available at www.humanmetrics.com. When you identify your four-letter code, read a chapter in the book, *Do What You Are*, describing key talents related to your profile (Tieger & Tieger 1995). The book is available in most of the larger public libraries. Another resource that addresses elders' strengths related to Jung's typology is *Creative Aging: Discovering the Unexpected Joys of Later Life Through Personality Type*, by Nancy Bost Millner (Millner 1998). In addition, use a search engine like Google, type in your four-letter code, and you will be led to a wealth of information about your profile.

Finally, skills inventories and other valuable assessment instruments are yours to explore at no cost at many university Internet career centers. To find some of them, enter "transferable skills" in Google. Over time, by reflecting on all of this information, you may be able to construct at least a partial description of your vocational legacy.

Connecting With Others

As mentioned in Section 1, gerotranscendence research suggests that, while the quantity of relationships may decline in our later years, the quality of our people connections often expands.

The film *Harry and Tonto* is an excellent example. Seventy-five-year-old Harry Coombes and his cat, Tonto, embark upon a soul-filled journey driving through the U.S. countryside and connect with a number of fascinating people.

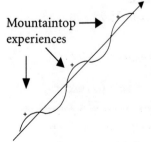

Mountaintop experiences

Bill Thomas underscores that elders have been engaged in important legacy-type activities in human communities for many centuries. First of all, they are peacemakers, and peacemakers heal conflict and our society. He is not alone in affirming society's desperate need for people who have outgrown violence and who can make peace in their families, communities, and in the world. Old people always have been the peacemakers, elders who have moved beyond the fevered desire to get and to hold on to power, leaving the world a better place for following generations as their legacy.

Living a legacy also includes connecting with others through the sharing of wisdom accumulated over many years of experience. Difficult to define, wisdom has to do with purposely applying knowledge and experience with common sense, insight, intelligence, feeling, and tolerance. We live in a time that cries out for solutions to daily issues; older adults offer many answers based upon their own experiences, if we but ask.

Another way of living a legacy by connecting to others involves giving unconditional positive regard through mentoring. Many of us remember a grandparent, teacher, aunt, or uncle who understood us when we were young and searching, giving us sound advice along the way. As opposed to parents who tend to be very task oriented, mentors are apt to be more relationship and process oriented. Concentration is focused upon "being with" as opposed to "doing for" a child.

Connecting with Everything: Cosmic Connectivity

A third way to engage your legacy as you age holistically includes exploring, expanding, and sharing one's spirituality and faith system. Again, according to Lars Tornstam's research on gerotranscendence, at this level of the aging process there tends to be an expanded understanding of the connectedness of everything.

Both Julia Riley and social worker Marty Richards affirm guiding elders to explore their personal strengths and to engage in life review, repair, and purpose. To that end, and as mentioned previously, we recommend a technique called *ethnographic interviewing*, one process to empower people and get to the narrative core of one's life. Some possible queries include:

- Describe what really makes a good day for you.
- If you were to visit a bookstore, what particular section would you find yourself drawn to? What titles interest you?
- What things do you do each day or this week through which you become totally absorbed?
- What in your life gives you the greatest possible joy?
- What life lessons have helped you cope throughout your years?
- Based upon your life experiences, what important message would you like to give to the world?
- At your memorial service, what would you like people to say about you as a way of summarizing your life and your gifts?

In varying ways, the three themes of connecting with self, others, and the cosmos surface in later life and contribute to creating and living your legacy. To highlight its vital importance, Rick Moody, editor of AARP's *Human Values in Aging* electronic newsletter, reports a conversation with Reb Zalman Schachter-Shalomi

(Moody 2005a). At one point Reb turned to him and said, "You know, there's really only one great question in life. It's the question, are you saved?" Rick was puzzled for a moment over what was meant, when Reb followed immediately by saying, "No, not in a theological sense, but in a computer sense." Reb Zalman was pointing to the question of legacy. Have we yet been "saved" in the sense of "downloading" our life experiences to the great "hard drive" of future generations, to those who will live after us?

References

Millner, N. 1998. *Creative Aging: Discovering the Unexpected Joys of Later Life Through Personality Type.* Palo Alto, CA: Davis-Black Publishing.

Moody, H.R. 2005a. AARP's *Human Values in Aging* E-mail Newsletter. aarpnews@news.aarp.org.

Bibliography

Armstrong, J. 1744. *The Art of Preserving Health.* http://www.giga-usa.com/quotes/authors/john_armstrong_a001.htm (accessed July 30, 2006).

Baltes, P.B., & J. Smith. 2003. New frontiers in the future of aging: From successful aging of the young old to the dilemmas of the Fourth Age. *Gerontology: Behavioural Science Section/Review* 49:123–35.

Berendt, J. 1983. *The World is Sound.* Rochester, UT: Destiny Books.

Bianchi, E. 1991. *Aging as a Spiritual Journey.* New York: Crossroad/Herder & Herder.

Brand, D. & P. Yancey. 1997. *The Gift of Pain.* Grand Rapids, MI: Zondervan Publishing.

Brhel, S. 2005. *Increasing the Quality of Life for the Older Adult.* Binghamton, New York: Brundage Publishing.

Buber, M. 1923. *I and Thou.* New York: Touchstone 1996 edition.

Burnside, I. 1986. *Working With the Elderly: Group Process and Techniques.* Boston: Jones and Bartlett.

Butler, R. 1969. Age-ism: Another form of bigotry. *The Gerontologist* 9:243–46.

Byock, I. 1997. *Dying Well: Peace and Possibilities at the End of Life.* New York: Riverside Books.

Callahan, M. & P. Kelley. 1992. *Final Gifts.* New York: Bantam Books.

Campbell, D. 2001. *The Mozart Effect.* New York: HarperCollins.

Carstensen, L., M. Pasupathi, U. Mayr, & J. Nesselroade. 2000. Emotional experiences in everyday life across the adult life span. *Journal of Personality and Social Psychology* 79(4):644–55.

Castillego, I. 1973. *Knowing Woman: A Feminine Psychology.* New York: Harper & Row.

Carter, J. 1998. *The Virtues of Aging.* New York: Ballantine Books, 1998.

Childs-Gowell, E. 1992. *Good Grief Rituals.* Barrytown, New York: Station Hill Press.

Clark, B. 1978. *Whose Life Is It?* New York: Avon Books.

Cohen, G. 2000. *The Creative Age: Awakening Human Potential in the Second Half of Life.* New York: Avon Books.

Cohen, G. 2005. *The Mature Mind.* New York: Basic Books.

Dass, R. 2000. *Still Here: Embracing Aging, Changing, and Dying*. New York: Riverside Books.

Deichman, E. & R. Kociecki. 1989. *Working With the Elderly: An Introduction*. Amherst, New York: Prometheus Books.

Dossey, B.M., L. Keegan, and C.E. Guzzetta. 2005. *Holistic Nursing: A Handbook for Practice*. 4th ed. Sudbury, MA: Jones and Bartlett, pp. 12–16.

Dossey, L. 1982. *Space, Time, and Medicine*. Boston: Shambhala.

Dychtwald, K. 1999. *Age Power: How the 21ˢᵗ Century Will Be Ruled by the New Old*. New York: Archer Putnam.

Erikson, E. *The Life Cycle Completed*. New York: W.W. Norton.

Feder, Judith. July-August 2005. "Do older Americans hide assets to qualify for Medicaid?" *Aging Today*, p. 9.

Fischer, K. 1998. *Winter Grace, Spirituality and Aging*. Nashville, TN: Upper Room.

Fourteen Friends. 1999. *Fourteen Friends' Guide to Eldercaring*. Sterling, VA: Capital Books.

Fox, M. 1983. *Original Blessing*. Santa Fe, NM: Bear and Co.

Friedan, B. 1993. *The Fountain of Age*. New York: Simon & Schuster.

Gambone, J. 2000. *Refirement: A Guide to Midlife and Beyond*. Minneapolis, MN: Kirk House Publishers.

Gentzler, R. Fall, 2005. "What do seniors want in a church?" *Center Sage* (newsletter). Nashville, TN: Center on Aging and Older-Adult Ministries.

Harkness, H. 1999. *Don't Stop the Career Clock*. Palo Alto, CA: Davies-Black.

Henry, L. & J. Henry. 1999. *Reclaiming Soul in Health Care*. Chicago: AHA Press.

Henry, L. & J. Henry. 2002. *The Soul of the Physician*. Chicago: AMA Press.

Henry, L. & J. Henry. 2004. *The Soul of the Caring Nurse*. Silver Springs, MD: Nursesbooks.org., the publishing arm of the ANA.

Hillman, J. 1999. *The Force of Character and the Lasting Life*. New York: Random House.

Hillman, J. 1996. *The Soul's Code*. New York: Random House.

Hooyman, N. & H. Kiyak. 2004. *Social Gerontology*. Boston: Allyn and Bacon.

Karnes, B. 2001. *Gone From My Sight – A Dying Experience*. Depoe Bay, OR: Barbara Karnes Books.

Kastenbaum, K. 2004. *Death, Society, and Human Experience*. Boston: Pearson Education, Inc.

Kataria, M. 2002. *Laugh for No Reason*. Mumbai, India: Madhuri International.

Kimble, M., ed. 2000. *Viktor Frankl's Contribution to Spirituality and Aging*. New York: Haworth Pastoral Press.

Kivnick, H. & S. Murray. 2001. Life strengths interview guide: Assessing elder clients' strengths. *Journal of Gerontological Social Work* 34(4):7–31.

Kliger, L. & D. Nedelman. 2006. *Still Sexy After All These Years? The 9 Unspoken Truths About Women's Desire After 50*. New York: Perigee/Penguin.

Kliger, L. and D. Nedelman. 2006. womenbeyond50.com (accessed July 30, 2006).

Kluger, J. January 16, 2006. "The Surprising Power of the Aging Brain." *Time Magazine* 167(3).

Kubler-Ross, E. 1969. *On Death and Dying*. New York: Touchstone.

LeDoux, J.E. 2002. *The Synaptic Self*. New York: Viking Penguin.

Leeds, J. 2001. *The Power of Sound*. Rochester, Vermont: Healing Arts Press.

Leslie, D.L., Y. Zhang, S.T. Bogardus, T.F. Holford, L. Leo-Summers, & S.K. Inouye. 2005. Consequences of preventing delirium in hospitalized older adults on nursing home costs. *Journal American Geriatric Society* 53:405-9.

Levoy, G. 1997. *Callings: Finding and Following an Authentic Life*. New York: Harmony Books.

Lustbader, W. and N. Hooyman. 1994. *Taking Care of Aging Family Members: A Practical Guide*. New York: Free Press.

Martz, S., ed. 1987. *When I Am an Old Woman I Shall Wear Purple*. Manhattan Beach, CA: Papier-Maché Press.

McLeod, B., ed. 2002. *And Thou Shalt Honor: The Caregiver's Companion*. New York: Rodale.

Millner, N. 1998. *Creative Aging: Discovering the Unexpected Joys of Later Life Through Personality Type*. Palo Alto, CA: Davis-Black Publishing.

Moody, H.R. March 2005a. AARP's *Human Values in Aging* E-mail Newsletter. aarpnews@news.aarp.org.

Moody, H.R., ed. 2005b. *Religion, Spirituality and Aging: A Social Work Perspective*. Binghamton, NY: Haworth Social Work Practice Press.

Morgan, R. 1996. *Remembering Your Story: A Guide to Spiritual Autobiography*. Nashville: Upper Room Books.

Needleman, J. 1985. *The Way of the Physician*. San Francisco: Harper & Row.

Palmer, P. 1999. *Let Your Life Speak*. San Francisco: Jossey-Bass.

Palmore, E., L. Branch, & D. Harris, eds. 2005. *Encyclopedia of Ageism*. New York: Haworth Pastoral Press .

Pipher, M. 1999. *Another Country: Navigating the Emotional Terrain of our Elders*. New York: Riverhead Books.

Rain, M. 2002. *Love Never Sleeps: Living at Home With Alzheimer's*. Charlottesville, VA: Hampton Roads.

Raines, R. 1998. *A Time to Live: Seven Steps of Creative Aging*. New York: Plume Printing.

Rantz, M. & M. Flesner. 2004. *Person-Centered Care*. Silver Springs, MD: American Nurses Association's Nursesbooks.org.

Rantz, M., L. Popejoy, & M. Zwygart-Stauffacher. 2001. *The New Nursing Homes*. Minneapolis: Fairview Press.

Ronch, J. & J. Goldfield. 2003. *Mental Wellness in Aging: Strength-Based Approaches*. Baltimore: Health Professions Press.

Roszak, T. 1998. *America The Wise: The Longevity Revolution and the True Wealth of Nations*. New York: Houghton Mifflin.

Roszak, T. 2001. *Longevity Revolution: As Boomers Become Elders.* New York: Warner Books.

Rowe, J and R. Kahn. 1998. *Successful Aging.* New York: Dell Publishing.

Sauer, R. Fall, 2005. "Senior adult spirituality group." *Center Sage* (newsletter). Nashville, TN: Center on Aging and Older-Adult Ministries.

Schachter-Shalomi, Z. 1995. *From Age-ing to Sage-ing: A Profound New Vision of Growing Older.* New York: Warner Books.

Schwartz, M. 1996. *Morrie: In His Own Words.* New York: Delta.

Simon, S. & S. Simon. 1991. *Forgiveness: How to Make Peace With Your Past and Get On With Life.* New York: Warner Books.

Singh, K. 2000. *The Grace in Dying: A Message of Hope, Comfort, and Spiritual Transformation.* New York: HarperCollins.

Snowdon, D. 2001. *Aging With Grace.* New York: Bantam.

Steindl-Rast, D. 1984. *Gratefulness, the Heart of Prayer: An Approach to Life in Fullness.* Ramsey, NJ: Paulist Press.

Tathagatannda, S. 2004. *Four Stages of Life.* New York: Vedanta Society of New York. http://www.vedanta-newyork.org/articles/vedanta101_7.htm (accessed July 30, 2006).

Taylor, D. 1997. *Biomedical Foundations of Music as Therapy.* St. Louis: MMB Music, Inc.

Thomas, W. 2004. *What Are Old People For?* Acton, MA: VanderWyk & Burnham.

Tieger, P. and B. Tieger. 1995. *Do What You Are.* Boston: Brown, Little.

Tornstam, L. 2005. *Gerotranscendence.* New York: Springer Publishing Company.

Vaillant, G. 2002. *Aging Well: Surprising Guideposts to a Happier Life.* Boston: Little, Brown.

Wadensten, B. and M. Carlsson. 2002. Theory-driven guidelines for practical care of older people, based on the theory of gerotranscendence. *Journal of Advanced Nursing* 36(5):635–42.

Willingham, R. 2003. *Hey, I'm the Customer.* Upper Saddle River, NJ: Prentice Hall.

Index

A

AACN. *See* American Association of Colleges of Nursing
achievement model, 12–13
action research, xvii
active imagination, 150
activities, formal programs, 70
activity, 17, 81, xviii
    as busyness, 132–133
acupuncture, 149
Acute Care for the Elderly (ACE) Units, 102
adaptability to change, 8–9
adoption, 163–164, xx
adult day health care, 84, 85–86, 87, xx
adult family homes, 90, 92
advocacy, 46, 114
age-specific care, 41
ageism, 7–10, 179
aging, 3, 5, 14, 21, 132
    dimensions, 136
    holistically, 139
    physiological, 108
    process, 31, 129, xv
aging in place, 113, 163
Aging Initiative, xviii
aging population, 54, 107
alternative and complementary medicine, 149
American Association of Colleges of Nursing (AACN), 99–100
archetypes, 16
art therapy, 82
assessment instruments, 184
autobiographies, 129
Ayurvedic system, 49, xxii

B

baby boomers, 6, 25, 157–158
bedside time, 41
being, 16–19, 20, 170, 180
BenefitsCheckUp program, 116
Bianchi, Eugene, 180
brain capabilities, 9
Bridge system, 41
Buchanan Place, 84–85, xx
Buddhist spirituality, 133–134
Building Academic Geriatric Nursing Capacity (BAGNC), 98, 99

C

callings, 124
care coordination, 53
care strategies, 164
caregivers, 86, 114, 153. *See also* nurses
    bedside time, 41
    coordinating services, 53, 60
    encouraging holistic services, 122
    family members, 143
    interacting with elders, 108, 146
    knowledge of aging process, 31
    music effects, 170
    personal healing, 158
    preparing for death, 124
    quality time, 128
    stress, 87
    support, 55–56
Center for Aging and Older Adult Ministries, xx
chaplains, 124–125
children and intergenerational issues, 74, 81

Chinese medicine, 65
choices, patients, 51, 52, 115, 144, 145
Christianity, 113, 121, 152, 162
    See also Good Samaritan Society;
        spirituality
churches, 7, 13–14, 127, 128–129
cognitive decline, 9, 36, 105, 162, 170. *See also*
        dementia
    risk factors for, 38
    spirituality and, 127–130
communication, 105, 128, 145
communities for elders and eldercare, 56,
        67–93, xx
    creating, 69, 71
    See also Elden Alternative; ElderHealth
        Northwest; Kendal at Ithaca;
        Sherbrooke Community Centre;
        TigerPlace
Community Options Program Entry System,
        85
complementary and alternative medicine, 149
Comprehensive Community Hospice, 46, 49
connections, 23, 150, 169, 184–185
Constant Source Seminars©, 156
consumer information, xxi
continuum of care, gaps, 43
contributions of elders, 22, 56, 100, 165
cosmetic industry, xv
cosmetic surgery, 7, 64
costs of medical care, evaluation models, 32
cultural death traditions, 173
culture, keepers of, 23
curriculum, 99, 102–104, 107, 115
customer service, 74

D
death, 83, 121, 173
    acceptance, 134, 161–162
    after-death traditions, 121–122
    facilitating a good death, 138
    preparations (*See* preparing for death)
decision-making, 51, 115, 144
Delirium. *See* dementia; cognitive decline
delirium, 33, 36, 38
    See also dementia; cognitive decline
dementia, 3–4, 65, 170
    interventions, 60
    patients living longer, 46–47
    See also cognitive decline
depression, 65

diagnostic strategies, 32
diminishment model, 11, xv
disassociation, 136
discharge planning, 31
discrimination, 86, xiv
    HIV/AIDS, 175
diversity of elders, 8
doing, 16–19, 133–134
dying process, 48, 70–71
    stages, 134
    See also preparing for death
dying workshops, 152–153
dying, working with, 139
dysmorphic disorder, 64

E
Eastern medicine, 149
Eastern spirituality, 133–134, 178
economic impact of aging population, 6
economic impact of elder participation, 13
Eden Alternative™, 19–20, 79, xx
    Klein Center, 74, 75
education, 59. *See also* curriculum
ego, 133
ego integrity, xv
elder abuse, 34, 65
elder communities/places, xx
Elder Friends, 88
eldercare, 67, 180–181, xxii
    baby boomer impact, 25
ElderHealth Northwest, 84
elders, 15, 19, 120, 122, xiv
    adoption of, 163–164
    as peacemakers, 23, 184
    as teachers, 111
    capacity for growth, 180
    contributions, 22, 56, 100, 165
    family support, 62
    leaving home, 130, 146
    societal regard, 119
    strengths, 180
emergency medicine, 29. *See also* geriatric
    emergency medicine
emotional system, 24, 63–64
employee motivation and retention, 116
employee stress, 87
end-of-life issues, 48, 138. *See also* legacy
    choices, 51, 52, 144
    initiating discussion, 162
    planning, 150

environment, 40, 85, 115, 164, 165
environmental press, 54
Ethical Wills, xxi
ethnographic interviewing, 185, xx
Evergreen Health Care (spiritual care), 152–155
exercise, 79, 82
expectations, aging, 21
expressive arts technique, 158, 159

F
falls, 37, 40
faith and aging, 124, 173
faith traditions. *See* religion
family care, 58, 160
family caregivers, 3–4, 105, 143
  sandwich generation, 153
family dynamics, 58, 59, 146
family support for elders, 62
financial resources, 4–5
financing long-term care, 75
Finding Meaning in Medicine, 56, xx
forgiveness, 137, 157
fulfillment, 23, 73, 79, 185
functional decline due to hospital care, 36–37, 39
funding for facilities, 88, 114
Future of Retirement research, 12

G
generativity, 176
geriatric consultation model, 37
geriatric education, 102–104
geriatric emergency medicine, 29, 30, 33, 34
geriatric nursing model, 110
Geriatric Resource Nurse (GRN), 102, xx
geriatrics, 39, 98
gerontophobic fear, 7, 179
gerotranscendence, 20–21, 72, 135, xv, xxii
  contributions of elders, 22
  creating conducive environment, 164
  elder strengths, 180
  guidelines, 146–147
  individual growth, 24–25
God. *See* spirituality
Good Samaritan Society, 113, 115
Greenhouse, xx
ground of being, 22
growth, elders' capacity for, 9, 180

H
Hartford Institute. *See* John A. Hartford Foundation Institute for Geriatric Nursing
Harvard Adult Study of Adult Development, 12, 14, xxii
healing modalities, 63, 149
health care, 17–18, 102
healthcare providers, 37, 41. *See also* caregivers; nurses
Hebrew Home for the Aged (HHAR), 34
HELP. *See* Hospital Elder Life Program
Hindu spirituality, 134
HIV/AIDS, 174–176
holism, embracing, 23–24
holistic approach, 18
holistic care, 57, xvi
  nursing therapies, 16
  reducing medications, 63
home care, safety, 113
home health model, 78
Honor My Wishes (end-of-life program), 52, xxi
hope, aspects of, 130
hopelessness, 62
hospices, 49, 162
  admission indicators, 47
  breaking even financially, 160–161
Hospital Elder Life Program (HELP), 36–39, xx
hospitals, 38, 101–102
  after care, 44
  discharge planning, 30
  functional decline, 36–37, 39
Housing and Urban Development (HUD) housing, 115

I
I and Thou, 120, 169
immobilization in hospital care, 37
Improving Care Through the End of Life, 51, xx
inclusivity, 124
individuality, 70, 72, 85
individuation, xv
institutionalization, 5, 72
intergenerational programming, 81
intergenerational relationships, 74
interventions, 60
isolation, social, 86

J

John A. Hartford Foundation Institute for Geriatric Nursing, 98, 99, 101, 103, xx
Judaism, 119, 121–122, 129

K

Kendal at Ithaca (elder community), 80
Klein Center (eldercare facility), 73
Kubler-Ross, Elizabeth, 134, 136

L

laughter, 154
Law of Manu (Hinduism), 133
learning environment, 115
legacy, personal, 116, 129, 159, 183
    connectivity, 185
    expressing, 158
leisure model, 11–12
life expansion, 11
life plans, callings, 124
life purpose, 23, 73, 79, 185. *See also* reason
        to live
life repair, 157, 185
life review, 156, 183–184, 185
life spans, 8
life-contingency planning, 144–145
lifting, 116
listening, 61
Living History Program, 73, xx
living in the present, 139
lobbying, 114
location of elder facilities, 81
long-term care, 4, 43, 72
    facility funding, 88
    Hartford Institute recommendations, 104
Lucerne Hospital, 124

M

Magnet (hospital) facilities, 40, 42
Make A Wish foundation, 116
manual lymph drainage, 149–150
media portrayal of elders, 15, xiv
Medicaid projections, 4
Medicare payment rate, 88
Medicare volunteer requirements, 161
medication reconciliation, 34, 41, 63, 79
memory abilities, 9
Mercy Health Center, 40
methodology, xvi

miracles, 125
mobility, 60, 79
    hospital care, 37
models of aging, 10–14
Montgomery hospice, 160–161
mortality feelings, 125
movies/videos, xxi
music practitioner, 167
music therapy, 82, 168–169, xxii
    caregivers, 170
Myers-Briggs Type Indicator®, 184, xxii

N

Nambudripad's Allergy Elimination
        Technique (NAET), 65
negative attitude of healthcare providers, 37
neuro-emotional complexes (NECs), 63
Neuro-Emotive Technique (NET), 63–64,
        xxii
Nurse Competence in Aging Project (NCA),
        102
nurses and nursing, 40–42, 50–51, 158
    education and training, 97, 103, 107
    geriatric, 44–45, 98
    hospice, 46–48
    psychiatric, 62, 65, 163
Nurses Improving Care to Health-system
        Elders Program (NICHE), 102, 110–
        111, xx
nursing crisis, 97
nursing curriculum, 99, 102–104
nursing homes, 49, 69, 78
    negative perceptions, 77
    practicing religion, 127–128
nursing standards, 101

O

OH Cards, 82, xxii
old age, definition of, 29, 30
    perceptions of, 6, 106

P

pastoral care, 41, 124
    dying and, 136–139
patient satisfaction with government
        reimbursement, 75
peacemaking, 23, 184
perception of time and space, 150
perceptions of aging, xiii–xiv

perceptions of elders, 179
perceptions of old, 6, 106
performance, positive impact factors, 19
pets, 71
phases of aging, 13
Philippines, the, 62
philosophy of aging, 20–21
physical environment accommodations, 40
physician education, 57
physician extenders, 43
Pioneer Network, 21, xx
political advocacy, 114
polypharmacy, 34, 41, 63, 79
post-hospital care, 44
prayer, 125, 139, 150
preparing for death, 24, 124, 138–139, 153
    comfort of religion, 173
    decision-making, 51
presence, connectivity, 169
PrestigePLUS, 148, xx
preventive care, 32
productivity, 132–134
Programs of All-inclusive Care for the
        Elderly, 116, xx
programs, strategies and resources, xx–
        xxiii

Q
Quality Improvement Program for Missouri,
    78
quality time, 128

R
reality orientation, 60
reason to live, 20. *See also* life purpose
receptivity, 17, 22–23, 170–171
reimbursement for long-term care, 75
reinvention in later life, 12
relationships, 70, 71, 73–74, 75
    quality of, 23
religion, 14, 127–128, 173. *See also* Christianity;
    Judaism; Good Samaritan Society;
        spirituality
reminiscence therapy, 82
resources, 104, xx–xxiii
respite self-care, 55
restraining patients, 40
retirement, 6, 12
retirement communities, 81

right to die, 151
rituals, 137

S
safety, home care, 113
sage-ing, 14, 156
sandwich generation, 153
scholarship program, 98–99
Second Journey, 25, xx
self-acceptance, 22
self-care, 55–56, 173
    elder abuse, 65–66
    strategies, 61
self-healing capacities, 168
senescence, 183
senility as cognitive decline, 9. *See also* cognitive
        decline
services, 53, 59, 60, 61
sexuality, 10
shadow, human, 22
Sherbrooke Community Centre, 69, 71–72
singing bowls, 172
sound, 167
spinal cord injuries, 44
spiritual eldering, 157
spiritual growth model, 13–14
spiritual support for caregivers, 55
spirituality, 59, 130, 139, xvii, xviii
    after-death traditions, 121–122
    Eastern insights, 133, 178
    feeling of mortality, 125
    holistic view, 123
    I and Thou, 120
    meeting needs, 75
    relationship with God, 119, 120
    religion, 14, 127–128, 173
    tasks of aging, 129
    See also Evergreen Health Care
Stephen minister and ministry, 152
stereotypes, 7–10, 15, 21, 75, xiv
storytelling, 150, 154
    written, 74, 155
strategies (overview), xx–xxiii
strengths-based, xvi
stringing beads (therapeutic), 159, xxii

T
T'ai Chi, 149, xxii
techniques in eldercare (overview), xxii

terminal restlessness, 137
terms for elders, 5, 7
Therapeutic Touch, 169, xxii
therapy and therapies 16, 82, xxii
    art therapy, 82
    laughter as, 154
    nursing therapies, 16
    music therapy, 82, 168–169, 170
    Neuro-Emotive Technique (NET), 63–64
    overview of, xxii
    reminiscence therapy, 82
    singing bowls, 172
    stringing beads, 159
    Therapeutic Touch, 169
    Thought Field Therapy, 61
    visionary therapy, 48
thinking function, 18
Thought Field Therapy, 61, xxii
TigerPlace (aging-in-place community
    concept), 5, 77–79
Time Slips, 159, xxii
time, redefinition of, 24
Tornstam, Lars, 20–21, 22, 180
touch drawing, 158–159

training, 41, xviii, xxi
    nurses, 97, 103, 107
transitioning decisions, 144
Transition Program, 53, 54, xx
transportation in emergencies, 100
trust, 172
turnover rate, 87

U
universal worker, 114

V
vibration, 167
visionary therapy, 48
volunteers, 38, 161
    Elder Friends, 88
    elder participation, 11, 83
    house calls, 52

W
wellness program, 148
Windhorse model, 164–165
workshops, xxi
worthiness, 133–134